21st Century Imaging

Quintessentials of Dental Practice – 28
Imaging – 3

21st Century Imaging

By

Keith Horner
Nicholas Drage
David Brettle

Editor-in-Chief: Nairn H F Wilson
Editor Imaging: Keith Horner

Quintessence Publishing Co. Ltd.
London, Berlin, Chicago, Paris, Milan, Barcelona, Istanbul,
São Paulo, Tokyo, New Delhi, Moscow, Prague, Warsaw

British Library Cataloguing in Publication Data

Horner, Keith
   21st century imaging. - (Quintessentials of dental practice; v. 28)
   1. Teeth - Radiography
   I. Title II. Drage, Nicholas III. Brettle, David
   617.6'07572

ISBN: 9781850970972

Copyright © 2008 Quintessence Publishing Co. Ltd., London

ISBN: 978-1-85097-097-2

Foreword

Diagnostic imaging is the commonest form of clinical investigation used in oral diagnosis. In contrast to what existed in the last quarter of the 20th century, practitioners now have a bewildering choice of imaging systems for use in everyday clinical practice. Imaging in the 21st century – Volume 28 in the unique *Quintessentials of Dental Practice* series, provides excellent insight and authoritative guidance on the use of contemporary imaging systems. As expected of titles in the *Quintessentials* series, this book has been carefully prepared to appeal to, in particular, busy practitioners and students at all levels. The text is generously illustrated, with each chapter concluding with carefully selected references or helpful suggestions for further reading.

With the prospect of different forms of digital imaging being widely used, if not largely replacing traditional diagnostic imaging in clinical practice in a matter of five to ten years, existing and future practitioners need to get to grips with the relevant technologies and clinical techniques as soon as is practically possible. This book provides the means to meet this challenge, with lots to interest and information for all members of the dental team. As has come to be expected of all volumes in the *Quintessentials* series, this is a read-in-a-few-hours, and then keep-to-hand book of immediate practical relevance. This book is a great addition to the *Quintessentials* series, which continues to go from strength to strength. It is a privilege and honour to be Editor-in-Chief of the series, helping to make books such as this volume available to busy colleagues across the world.

Nairn Wilson
Editor-in-Chief

Preface

The 20th century saw a slow, steady evolution in dental x-ray imaging. Despite obvious improvements in the quality and sophistication of equipment and materials for dental radiography over the first hundred years after Roentgen's discovery of x-rays, the basic photographic based technologies are the direct descendents of those used in the 1890s. In the 21st century, the foot has been put firmly down on the accelerator as far as dental imaging is concerned. Digital imaging is rapidly becoming the method of choice for dentists in many countries and now we are faced with exciting new developments that promise to revolutionise the way we use images to help in managing our patients.

In writing this book, we had in mind the dentist who was looking for information about "state of the art" dental imaging. While commencing with some historical information to set the scene, we decided to concentrate particularly on digital imaging. Thus, three chapters are devoted specifically to this subject. Nonetheless, despite a "high tech" emphasis in much of the book, we have still included information on conventional image receptors; film remains a cheap and adequate way of imaging dental patients that should not be consigned to the history books just yet. We have also included information on intra oral and panoramic equipment, to help the reader understand what is available and the ideal features to seek when buying. In the final chapter, "Implant Imaging" we have focused on the more complex imaging techniques and equipment that a dentist is unlikely to consider buying, but for which he or she may refer patients.

Keith Horner

Acknowledgements

We thank our families, friends and colleagues for their encouragement and support while writing this book.

Contents

Chapter 1

The Historical Perspective

Aim

The aim of this chapter is to provide an historical perspective for the current developments in dental x-ray imaging.

Outcome

The reader will have knowledge of the earliest use of x-rays in dentistry and of the subsequent developments, setting the scene for the important developments in dental imaging in the early years of the 21st century.

The First Steps

Dentists first made radiographs of their patients in the early months of 1896, within weeks of the 1895 publication of Röntgen's discovery of x-rays. It is difficult to say exactly who produced the first dental radiograph, but it is certain that at least four individuals were independently experimenting with x-rays in the oral cavity: Walkhoff (Fig 1-1) and Koenig in Germany, Kells in the USA and Harrison in England. Frank Harrison is of particular interest for two reasons. First, because he carefully recorded his work and published this in the *Journal of the British Dental Association* in June 1896; second, because his radiographs were of acceptable clinical quality (Fig 1-2).

How was it done? Harrison's records show that, in the absence of a mains electrical supply, radiography needed substantial battery power. To this was added a transformer (homemade) to produce high voltages; finally, he used a hand-crafted glass x-ray tube. An example of such an installation is shown in Fig 1-3. In these respects he was simply following the methods of Röntgen. Such equipment was unreliable in its output and was constantly subject to breakdown. A further challenge was the means of recording an image. Following Röntgen's own method, Harrison initially used photographic glass plates, cut down to size and wrapped in rubber dam, but he soon switched to "Eastman's Kodac" [sic] film. With this apparatus and material, he was able to produce radiographs with 6-minute exposures.

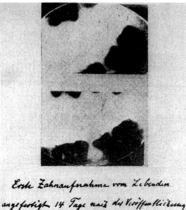

Fig 1-1 One of the first radiographs of teeth, taken by Otto Walkhoff in Germany in the early months of 1896.

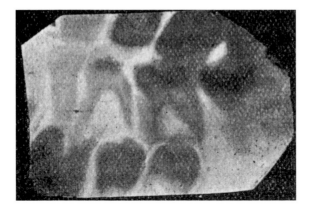

Fig 1-2 Dental radiograph of a 7-year-old girl taken by Frank Harrison in Sheffield in 1896. The exposure time was several minutes.

Harrison was among the earliest to report radiation injuries. He reported practising his techniques on his male assistant, who was acting as a patient, over a four-week period in 1896. The consequences were dramatic:

On June 4 the patient complained of an itching and burning sensation, with slight redness over the area subjected to the x-rays; shaving had to be discontinued on account of pain.... On the 6th the hair follicles of the beard and right side of the moustache appeared to postulate. On June 8 ... the skin commenced to desquamate; on the next day the hair over the affected region began to fall... The hair has continued to fall up to the date of writing (June 24), and the skin of the face is quite bald, and the glossy skin in slight wrinkles.

Journal of the British Dental Association (1896)

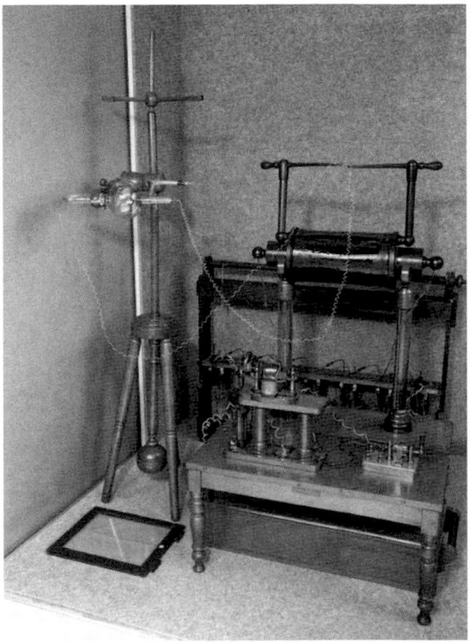

Fig 1-3 An x-ray installation from 1896/97. On the left is the x-ray tube and on the right is the electrical apparatus required to produce the electrical supply. (Courtesy of the Science Museum, London).

In most respects, Harrison's report was a microcosm of the collective experiences of early pioneers of dental radiography: ramshackle collections of x-ray generating equipment, homemade adaptations of photographers' materials and sporadic radiation-induced injuries. It was a faltering start to x-ray imaging in dentistry and it is unsurprising that Harrison ended his paper with the statement: "the work is altogether too complicated and too expensive to be added to the dental outfit".

Progress in X-ray Equipment

The early years of the 20th century saw rapid improvements in medical x-ray generating equipment. Within months of Röntgen's discovery, several scientists had independently developed a "focus tube". In simple terms, this moved the anode of the x-ray tube from a position perpendicular to the electron beam to one at an angle, leading to a smaller source of the x-rays (and hence sharper images) and a longer tube life.

3

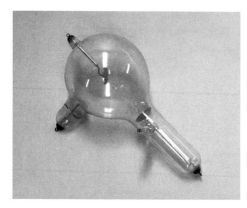

Fig 1-4 This early x-ray tube shows the additional side protuberance, which allowed "regulation" of the tube to keep it working optimally.

Early x-ray tubes, far from being evacuated, contained a lot of air. Indeed, in the beginning this air was essential to provide an electron source for x-ray production. These tubes were highly unpredictable in operation: during use the vacuum improved, but it then deteriorated when the tube was idle. To deal with this challenge, tubes had small projections in the glass bulb that contained a screw cap (Fig 1-4); this cap could be briefly opened to allow a little air to enter, thus restoring tubes that had been used heavily and had too high a vacuum. This "hit and miss" x-ray production meant that the operator was forced to test the x-ray output frequently, usually on himself or an unfortunate assistant. The process of "setting the tube" stored up many future problems in terms of delayed radiation injuries and cancer induction.

Mains electrical supply was far from universal at the start of the 20th century. Instead, power supplies were limited to pulsating direct voltage from induction coils, with the reverse currents (anode to cathode) giving poor efficiency and shortening tube life. The introduction of transformers and AC mains supplies in the first and second decades of the 20th century improved the situation substantially. The key development, however, was the patenting of the "hot cathode" x-ray tube by Coolidge in 1913 (Fig 1-5). Coolidge used a tungsten filament as the cathode and a good vacuum was achievable, allowing a vastly superior efficiency of x-ray production. Although numerous modifications were made over the subsequent years, this invention is the real ancestor of the x-ray tube found in modern x-ray machines, including dental sets.

In the early years, dentists simply copied medical equipment, putting together components bought at the local chemists or hardware store or by mail order.

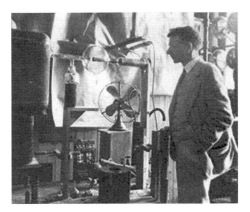

Fig 1-5 William Coolidge in his laboratory, with an example of his "hot cathode" x-ray tube.

It was not until 1905 that the first "dental x-ray set" was manufactured in Germany, followed in 1912/13 by two US manufacturers. Early x-ray equipment had exposed high-voltage wires, which were a serious danger to the operator; indeed, the risk of electrocution was as serious as that of x-ray injury. In 1918, the first shockproof dental x-ray set was introduced in the USA. The Victor CDX used an oil-filled container to house the x-ray tube and electrical wires, a method of insulation that is still used today. Nonetheless, equipment with exposed wiring continued to be used for some years.

Thus, the basics of a safe and efficient x-ray machine for dentists were in place by the 1920s. By the next decade, designs incorporating the new streamlined art deco style were being produced (Fig 1-6), with a position-

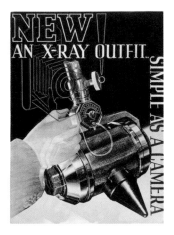

Fig 1-6 An advertisement for a state-of–the-art dental x-ray set from the 1930s. Note the pointed cone to aid in positioning during radiography. (Courtesy of the Science Museum, London).

5

indicator cone to aid in radiographic positioning. Such equipment had a long life, and older dentists may even remember sets like this persisting beyond the middle of the century.

While the revolution in dental x-ray set design was complete, certain developments were still to come though a slower and more evolutionary process. One important change was the introduction of electronic rather than clockwork timers, a change that was essential to cope with the shorter exposure times achievable with faster films. The "pointed cone" position indicating device seen in Fig 1-6 was gradually displaced by open-ended cylinders during the 1970s, reducing scatter and clearly demarcating the irradiated area. In the last decade of the 20th century, constant-potential x-ray equipment gradually became available to dentists, shortening exposure times and avoiding the "pulsating" x-ray production associated with mains voltage.

One key development in dental radiography in the 20th century was "panoramic imaging". The full story has been told in Chapter 1 of *Panoramic Radiology* (Quintessentials of Dental Practice – 20; Imaging – 2, 2006) and the reader is referred there for information. Briefly, however, early attempts to produce panoramic images of the jaws can be traced back to 1922. Panoramic imaging using intraoral x-ray sources was tried in the 1940s and early 1950s, but it gave poor image quality and very high radiation doses to the mouth. What we now recognise as panoramic radiography was developed in the 1940s by the Finnish scientist Yrjö Veli Paatero, who built on previous ideas of other researchers (Fig 1-7). Paatero employed a slit-collimated x-ray beam and a film cassette, with relative movement of these and the patient

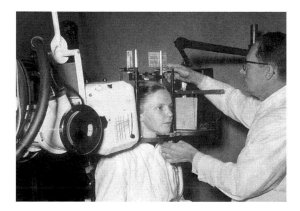

Fig 1-7 Dr Paatero making fine adjustments to patient positioning. The device was subsequently installed in Helsinki University in 1951. (Kindly supplied by Instrumentarium Imaging, Tuusala, Finland).

producing a scan image of the jaws. From early machines with single rotation centres, developments included increasing the number of centres to three and, more recently, to a continuously moving centre of rotation. Today, panoramic equipment offers several sophisticated options, including imaging of selected areas and cross-sectional imaging for implantology.

Progress in Image Receptors

Roll photographic film was the choice of early dental radiography practitioners, and this method persisted for two decades. Although one manufacturer produced ready-wrapped film in 1913, most dentists persisted with preparing films on an individual patient basis. It would not be until 1919 that the very first machine-wrapped dental film was manufactured: Kodak "Regular" film. This, as much as developments in equipment, made radiography a more attractive proposition for consideration by the average dentist.

While film remained the main focus of radiography, the use of intraoral fluoroscopy should not be forgotten. This involved the use of an instrument that, ostensibly, looked like a dental mouth mirror (Fig 1-8) but which had a fluorescent material in place of the mirror. If this was placed in the mouth behind a tooth and exposed then a "real time" image would appear. Despite its "instant imaging" attractions, this technique led to excessive x-ray exposures, not least to the operator, as the temptation to keep the x-rays turned on was strong.

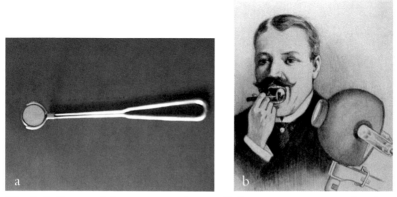

Fig 1-8 Intraoral fluoroscopy; a) a small fluorescent screen is fitted to a mouth mirror type handle; b) early drawing of this instrument in use.

7

In 1924, Kodak produced a double-sided film emulsion (Kodak "Radia-tized"), which halved the exposure times needed for imaging. Thereafter, developments were principally related to improving film speed. In 1940, "Ultraspeed" film allowed exposure times to be reduced by half. This was followed by further speed improvements in the 1950s. In the following decade, the polyester base was introduced, which was more robust than the cellulose acetate that had been in use since the 1930s. In 1980, "E-speed" film was introduced, once again halving the required exposure times, while in recent years we have seen a move to film speeds that fall into the "F-speed" category (see Chapter 4).

In 1989, there was a major development in dental radiography, with the first digital system for recording images: RadioVisioGraphy (Fig 1-9). This was developed by a French dentist, Francis Mouyen, and was based on a combination of the old fluoroscopy methods (Fig 1-8) with new video charged-couple device (CCD) camera technology. As with most clever inventions, the idea was simple: link a fluorescent screen to a video camera using some optical coupling. This combination was contained in a rather bulky sensor. Despite its primitive form and limitations, this development started the process of bringing dental radiography towards the 21st century. Today, there are many manufacturers of digital radiography equipment and a number of underlying technologies. These will be the focus of much of this book, notably in Chapters 5, 6 and 7.

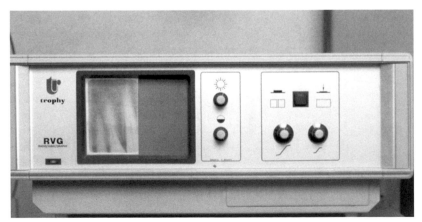

Fig 1-9 RadioVisioGraphy, the first digital dental radiography system, marketed in 1989.

Progress in Techniques

In the 1890s, dental radiography was a case of placing the glass plate or film where it would fit reasonably comfortably, placing the patient close to the x-ray tube, and hoping for the best while turning on the electrical supply. This method certainly produced images of teeth, but by no means could these images by described by our modern terminology of bitewing or periapical radiographs.

The first technique to be advocated was the positioning of the film parallel to the tooth and the central x-ray placed perpendicular to it: the "paralleling technique". This was described by Kells as far back as 1896, but was recognised more widely following publications by Price in 1904. Cieszynski, a Pole, developed the bisecting angle technique in 1907, whereby images of teeth could be produced by the principle of isometry. This required a "good eye" and a clear understanding of the technique, but it was facilitated in 1918 by the invention of an angle meter by the Indiana dentist Howard Raper. This device was subsequently incorporated into dental x-ray set design, and it can still be found on every intraoral machine. It was not until 1925 that Kells developed the bitewing technique, a technique that is as valuable today as ever it was.

While the paralleling technique was always the most obvious method of making periapical radiographs, it required clever positioning to ensure parallelism between film and tooth. Film-holding devices can be traced back to the very earliest years of dental radiography, with Harrison describing a stent fixed to his film and gripped between the teeth, a method also described by Kells in the USA and probably developed, using common sense, by most early dental radiographers.

Placing a film parallel to the tooth inevitably leaves a gap between the two. With a short distance between x-ray source and film, and the associated divergent beam, this can lead to marked magnification effects, with the image extending off the edge of the film, and anatomical distortion. This problem was addressed first by Franklin McCormick in San Francisco in 1910, who advocated a long source-to-film distance to improve the geometry. Promulgation of this method was continued by his son in the 1930s, while his son-in-law, Gordon Fitzgerald, developed the "long cone" in 1947. It is salutary to note that in many countries the very short ($\leq$ 10 cm) source-to-film distance has only recently been phased out of practice, despite its obvious image quality disadvantages. Along with the long-cone technique,

9

film-holding beam-aiming devices were devised to perfect technique, devices that are familiar to us today.

Progress in Radiation Safety

Harrison's early reports of radiation injuries associated with dental radiography were far from unique, with numerous case reports and vigorous discussion on the aetiology scattered throughout the dental literature of the time. In 1898, William Rollins, a dentist from Boston, USA, carried out animal tests which demonstrated that "X-ray light" could cause burns or even death. He is notable for his early recommendations for filtration of the x-rays to remove the low-energy radiation that causes skin damage and for his advice on the introduction of collimation and lead shielding. Sadly, many of his suggestions did not become accepted practice for many years. It is remarkable that Coolidge, whose new x-ray tube design did so much to improve medical radiology, should have referred extensively to Rollins' book *On X-ray Light*, published two decades previously.

Some pioneers in dental radiology, notably Kells, denied that x-ray exposure was strongly associated with disease and continued to opine this into the 1920s. It is ironic that Kells, who did so much to further the practice of dentistry, was ultimately to fall victim to severe radiation-induced injuries, including cancer, requiring as many as 100 operations and serial amputations.

Improvements in safety reflect factors related to the x-ray set and the image receptor. The steady rise in film speed has already been noted, providing a highly cost-effective means of dose reduction for patients. In terms of the x-ray set itself, the key events in improving safety were filtration, lead shielding and collimation, and the longer source-to-film distances. In terms of collimation, it should be remembered that early x-ray equipment offered nothing; the operator might be exposed to a considerable x-ray exposure, as might parts of the patient distant from the area of interest. By the 1930s, however, the shielded and collimated x-ray sets were overcoming this problem. Nonetheless, with short source-to-film distances the divergent beam meant that a considerable volume of patient could be exposed, even if the area on the skin covered by the beam was small. Collimation has steadily been improved over the years, to a standard of 6 cm diameter round beams in the 1970s, and more recently to rectangular collimation matching the normal size of dental intraoral film.

Concluding Comments

The path taken by dental radiography since 1896 can neatly be divided into four periods. First was the pioneering days between 1896 and the time of the Great War. This was the time of the amateur radiographer, struggling with unreliable equipment and materials. Only a few experts, such as Kells in the USA, mastered dental radiography, and it was seen as a rather unusual dental specialisation. The end of the Great War can be seen as a watershed, after which dental equipment and film began to be manufactured and electrical supplies became more readily available. A long period of evolution of equipment was associated with improved quality and safety, and an increasing proportion of dentists took up radiography. The third period can be traced from the 1950s and early 1960s, when panoramic radiography equipment was developed and first marketed. The final period began in 1989, with the first commercially available digital radiography system for dentists. In the 21st century we are faced with a bewildering array of digital equipment aimed at dentists and some exciting new developments such as cone-beam computed tomography. In the rest of this book we will explore what it takes to have "21st century imaging" in dental practice.

Further Reading

Rushton VE. Panoramic Radiography: History and Future Development. In: Rushton VE, Rout J. Quintessentials of Dental Practice 20 - Panoramic Radiology. London: Quintessence, 2006.

Chapter 2

Intraoral X-ray Equipment and Imaging

Aim

The aim of this chapter is to describe modern intraoral x-ray equipment, in particular those design features that improve safety and image quality.

Outcome

The reader should be able to:
- recognise the key features in modern intraoral x-ray equipment
- explain the safety design features of modern intraoral x-ray equipment
- explain how the design features of the x-ray set can affect image quality
- relate safety and image quality to current regulations and good practice guidelines.

Components of an Intraoral X-ray Set

Various components make up an intraoral dental x-ray set, the functions of which are shown in Table 2-1. A typical intraoral set is shown in Fig 2-1.

The X-ray Tube

The x-ray tube is composed of an evacuated glass tube containing a cathode (tungsten filament) and an anode (tungsten target set into a copper stem). A low current, typically around 7 mA, is passed through the tungsten filament, producing a cloud of electrons by thermionic emission. A focusing cup surrounding the filament keeps the electrons near to the filament. The electrons are then accelerated towards the tungsten target by the high potential difference (60–70 kV) between the cathode and the anode. The electrons are travelling fast when they strike the focal spot in the target and rapidly lose their kinetic energy in the form of heat and x-ray photons. The heat is conducted away from the tungsten target by the copper stem and is further dissipated by the surrounding oil. The x-ray photons pass through the thin glass tube. The components of the x-ray tube are shown in Fig 2-2.

Table 2-1 **Basic components of an intraoral dental x-ray set**

X-ray tube head	
Component	*Function*
X-ray tube	Site of x-ray production
Tube head housing	Metal casing that helps prevent leakage of radiation. It is filled with oil to help dissipate the heat generated during x-ray production
Step-up transformer	Steps up the voltage applied across the x-ray tube from 240 V to between 60-70 kV
Step-down transformer	Steps down the voltage applied to the filament to 10 V
Autotransformer	Allows the kV to be varied on those sets with variable kV selection
Aluminium filter	Filters out low-energy x-ray photons
Collimator	Metal component that defines the size and shape of the x-ray beam
Position indicating device (PID)	Device that allows the beam to be aimed accurately at the area under investigation and also sets up the focus-to-skin distance
Extension arm	
The arm allows precise and steady positioning of the x-ray tube head so that the position indicating device may be aligned correctly	
Exposure control panel and exposure button	
The panel allows the setting of the exposure time. The milliamperage (mA) is normally fixed by the manufacturer and is not adjustable. Some machines allow the operator to adjust the kV. Once the exposure factors have been set, pressing the exposure button activates the exposure.	

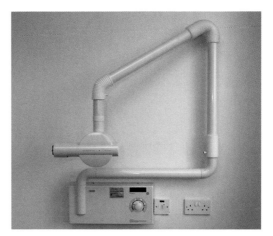

Fig 2-1 An example of a modern intraoral x-ray set.

a

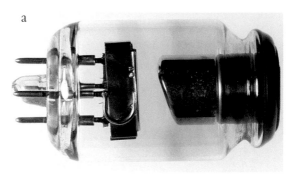

b

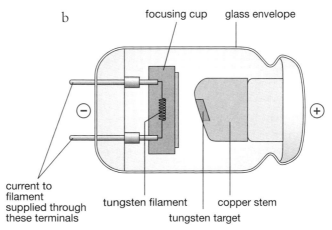

focusing cup   glass envelope

⊖   ⊕

current to
filament
supplied through   tungsten filament   copper stem
these terminals
tungsten target

Fig 2-2 a) The dental x-ray tube; b) The main components in the x-ray tube.

15

Recommendations for X-ray Equipment

In the UK, intraoral dental x-ray sets are designed and constructed so that they comply with British Standards and meet the safety and performance standards set out in the Medical Devices Regulations 1994. In the USA, all x-ray machines have to comply with performance standards set out by the Food and Drug Administration in 1995. Similar regulations are found in other countries.

Although the dose from one intraoral exposure is low, intraoral radiography is one of the commonest x-ray investigations undertaken in both the UK and USA. Therefore, the principle of "optimisation" should be followed at all times – keeping the radiation dose as low as reasonably practicable. Modern intraoral equipment incorporates many dose saving design features, the requirements for which include the following:
- New equipment should operate at a high kilovoltage.
- Constant potential units are superior to alternating current x-ray sets.
- The x-ray tube, x-ray housing and position indicating device should be constructed to keep radiation leakage to a minimum.
- Adequate filtration of the x-ray beam should be employed.
- Open-ended position indicating devices should be used in conjunction with rectangular collimation.
- The position indicating device should provide a long focus-to-skin distance.

Kilovoltage
The kilovoltage refers to the potential difference applied across the x-ray tube. Strictly speaking, the term "kV$_p$" (peak kilovoltage) should be used as this reminds us that the stated kilovoltage is that achieved at the peak of the alternating potential provided by the mains electrical supply. For simplicity, this book uses the term "kV". If a high kV is selected, the electrons in the x-ray tube are accelerated more and will be travelling more rapidly when they hit the target. The interaction of these electrons with the tungsten target will produce higher energy x-ray photons. Higher energy photons have shorter wavelength and are more penetrating. Therefore, these photons are less likely to get absorbed, decreasing the skin dose. A kV of between 60 and 70 kV is generally recommended.

However, the kV also has an effect on the quality of the image, in particular the radiographic contrast. The relationship between patient dose and radiographic contrast is discussed later.

Constant-potential Units

As indicated above, the mains power supply is alternating potential, and hence alternating current (AC). This means that the current is continuously oscillating from positive to negative. Each complete oscillation is known as a cycle. The number of cycles per second will vary depending on the country; there are 50 cycles per second (50 hertz) in the UK and 60 cycles per second (60 hertz) in the USA.

The mains voltage follows a similar waveform to the current (Fig 2-3). Only the positive half of the cycle is useful in producing x-rays. Rectification circuits ensure a positive kV is always applied across the tube.

- In full wave rectification, there are 100 pulses per second (in the UK), but peak voltage is only achieved for a short period of time. For the remaining time the kV is lower, producing lower energy x-ray photons. These lower energy photons increase the skin dose to the patient.
- Use of a three-phase rectification circuit ensures that the kV never falls to zero. The voltage waveform is a "ripple" rather than a pulse. The mean energy of the beam is increased, and so the dose to the patient is reduced.
- Constant-potential units have a continuously high voltage across the tube. This produces a beam with even higher mean energy and reduces the dose even further. Strictly speaking, the term "kV_{cp}" should be used for this type of equipment, where "cp" stands for constant potential. Because the output is more predictable in constant-potential units, they are a better choice for digital imaging systems.

If a constant-potential unit is used, the kV needs to be reduced to maintain the same radiographic contrast. For this reason the *European Guidelines on Radiation Protection in Dental Radiology* recommend 65–70 kV_p for AC equipment and 60 kV_{cp} for constant-potential units.

Radiation Leakage

The amount of leakage should be minimised to protect both the patient and the operator. Even though the housing is lined with metal, inevitably there will be some leakage of radiation. This is one of the reasons the operator should never stand inside the controlled area, or hold the x-ray tube head whilst making an exposure. In addition, the x-ray tube head should be strong and robust to ensure that if the tube head is knocked, the housing resists fracture.

Filtration

The x-ray photons originating from the target have a range of energies, with many low-energy and fewer high-energy photons generated. Aluminium

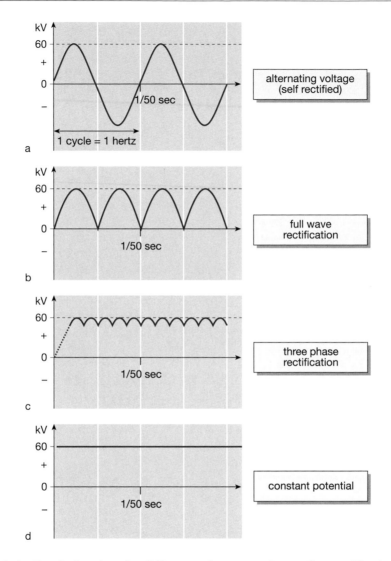

Fig 2-3 Graph showing the different voltage waveforms after rectification; a) Alternating voltage (self rectified), the voltage varies from positive to negative but x-rays are only produced when the voltage is positive; b) full wave rectification, there is no negative voltage across the tube but the voltage is still very variable; c) three phase rectification, the mean voltage still varies slightly (ripples) but the mean voltage across the tube is higher; d) constant potential, there is a constant high voltage across the tube.

filtration is used to filter out low-energy, longer wavelength x-ray photons, which would otherwise be absorbed in the patient's skin and not contribute to image formation. The more aluminium filtration that is used, the higher the mean energy of the x-ray beam. The skin dose to the patient is therefore dramatically reduced by the use of aluminium filtration. The amount of filtration required depends upon the kV of the x-ray set. It is generally accepted that for x-ray sets operating up to and including 70 kV the amount of filtration should be equivalent to not less than 1.5 mm of aluminium. For x-ray sets operating above 70 kV, more filtration is required. An aluminium filter is shown in Fig 2-4.

Rectangular Collimation
The advantage of using rectangular collimation is that it reduces the dose to the patient by at least 50% compared with standard 60 mm diameter round collimation. In the UK it is recommended that the rectangular collimation should not be larger than 40 x 50 mm. This ensures that it produces a suitable field size for use with the intraoral films in common use. In the USA, the recommendation is that the rectangular collimation should not exceed the dimension of the film by more than 2% of the focus-to-film distance. The size of the exposure field when rectangular collimation is used is shown in Fig 2-5.

When the volume of tissue irradiated is reduced there will be less scatter of the x-ray beam within the patient. This ensures improved image quality, since scattered x-ray photons that strike the film emulsion will degrade the

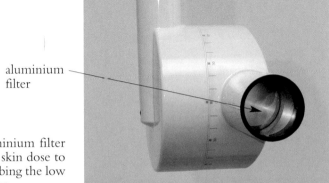

aluminium filter

Fig 2-4 The aluminium filter helps to reduce the skin dose to the patient by absorbing the low energy x-ray photons.

19

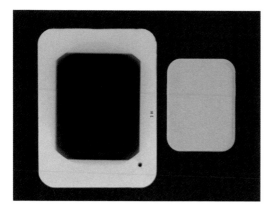

Fig 2-5 Size 4 (occlusal size) film irradiated using a rectangular collimator. This shows that the x-ray field is similar in size to that of a size 2 film packet.

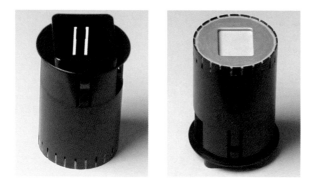

Fig 2-6 An example of a rectangular collimator that may be fitted into the circular position indicating device.

image. Reduced scatter is also beneficial to operators as it helps to reduce the radiation dose they receive.

New equipment can be purchased with rectangular collimation. If an existing x-ray set has open-ended round collimation then rectangular collimators can be retrofitted into the position indicating device (Fig 2-6). Some manufacturers produce "generic" rectangular collimators that can be fitted to any existing equipment.

In oblique lateral radiography, when the region of interest is often large, it is preferable to use round collimation to ensure the region of interest is covered. If round collimation is used, it is recommended the beam diameter at the end of the position indicating device should not exceed 60 mm (UK) or 70 mm (Canada).

Focus-to-skin Distance

The outer casing of the tube head should have the nominal focal spot marked. This indicates the source of x-ray production, known as the "focus". Hence it is easy to measure the distance between the focus and the skin, the focus-to-skin distance (fsd), as shown in Fig 2-7. A long fsd is recommended because it reduces the volume of tissue irradiated (Fig 2-8). In addition, the salivary glands, which are radiosensitive organs, are less likely to be included in the field. Using a long fsd may reduce the dose by up to 30%.

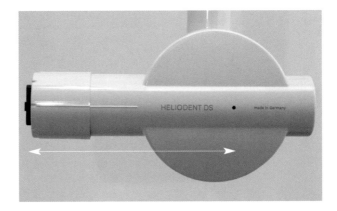

Fig 2-7 Nominal focal spot marked on the side of casing. This allows the fsd to be measured (arrowed line).

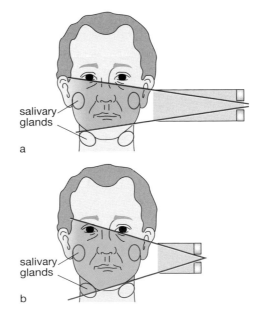

Fig 2-8 Diagram showing how altering the fsd affects the volume of tissue irradiated; a) long fsd, smaller volume of tissue irradiated; b) short fsd, larger volume of tissue irradiated. Also note that in this example, more salivary gland tissue is included in the field with a short fsd.

21

A long fsd automatically creates a long focus-to-tooth distance, which helps to improve image geometry. The longer the focus-to-tooth distance the more parallel the x-ray beam, and the less the image becomes magnified. The image is also sharper because the penumbra effect (edge unsharpness) is also reduced. This is explained in Fig 2-9.

In the UK it is recommended that the fsd is 200 mm for equipment operating at 60 kV or higher and at least 100 mm for equipment operating below 60 kV. In the USA the minimum recommended fsd is 200 mm, and in Canada the minimum acceptable fsd is 180 mm.

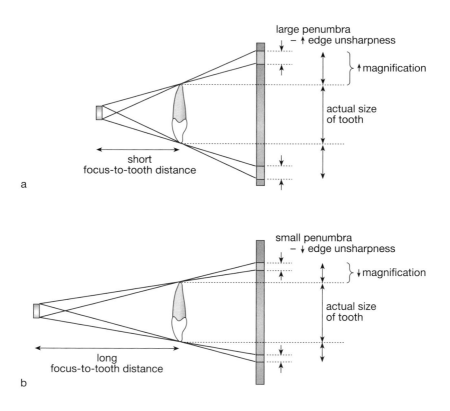

Fig 2-9 Diagram showing how altering the focus-to-tooth distance affects image quality; a) short focus-to-tooth distance, greater edge unsharpness and more magnification; b) long focus-to-tooth distance, less edge unsharpness and less magnification.

Other Important Features of Modern Dental X-Ray Sets

Focal Spot Size

Because of the penumbra effect, the larger the effective focal spot the greater the problem of image unsharpness. Consequently, a small filament is used, and the target is angled at about 20° to the electron source (Fig 2-10). This reduces the size of the effective focal spot to 0.5–1 mm.

Electronic Timers and Exposure Buttons

All modern x-ray sets have electronic timers that give accurate exposure times. The exposure button will only produce an exposure whilst continuous pressure is applied. If the pressure is released then the exposure terminates. The buttons are also designed to prevent immediate inadvertent re-exposure of the patient if the button is accidentally pressed again. The exposure buttons are located so that the operator can stand outside of the controlled area during the exposure. This is achieved by having the exposure button on a long expandable cable, or by wall mounting the control panel at a suitable distance from both the patient and the x-ray tube head. In the UK a minimum distance of 2 m is recommended, while in other countries, such as Canada, at least 3 m is recommended.

Exposure Factors

If a high kV is selected, the skin dose is lower because there is less absorption in the tissues. The resultant image, however, is of low contrast; it appears "flatter" as it contains many shades of grey. A low kV produces an image with high contrast, i.e. it contains fewer shades of grey and appears much more "black and white". This is because there has been more absorption within the tissues.

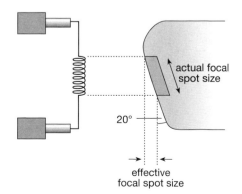

Fig 2-10 Diagram showing how using an angled target reduces the effective spot size. This in turn will help reduce edge unsharpness.

23

As well as being the main factor that determines contrast, kV also affects the density, or "blackening", of the image. Increasing the kV increases the density of the image because more x-ray photons are produced. Conversely, decreasing the kV reduces the density of the image. Therefore, if the kV is reduced in order to increase the contrast, then either the milliamperage (mA) or the time of the exposure must be increased to keep the density the same. Typically the mA is fixed, so it is normally necessary to adjust the time of the exposure.

Using a very high kV has a detrimental effect on the image contrast. For this reason a kV greater than 70 kV is not recommended for intraoral imaging. If a constant-potential unit is being used, a kV higher than 60 kV is not recommended, again because of the poor radiographic contrast.

On several new intraoral dental x-ray sets a choice of kV is available. Some authorities advocate the use of a lower kV if the primary objective is to identify caries, as this will produce greater contrast between the lesion and intact enamel or dentine. This is controversial as other authorities believe that if a higher kV is used, the increase in the number of shades of grey in the image will improve caries detection.

Alteration of the kV may be useful when managing large patients. As the tissues are thicker, more penetration of the tissues is required to produce the image, and so a higher kV should be selected.

A summary of the effects of altering exposure factors on image density and contrast is given in Table 2-2.

Aids to Intraoral Radiographic Technique

Intraoral radiography is an exacting skill and requires precision in placement of the film and in orientation of the x-ray beam. There are three common technique errors in intraoral radiography:
- incorrect film placement (Fig 2-11a)
- bending of the film (Fig 2-11b)
- incorrect alignment of the x-ray beam (Fig 2-11c).

These three problems are most effectively dealt with by use of a film-holding device that includes:
- a bite block to maintain correct film position
- a rigid backing to support the film and prevent bending
- an extraoral beam-aiming device to allow accurate alignment.

Table 2-2 **Effect of altering kV, mA and exposure time on image characteristics**

Variable	Change to variable	Effect on image	
		Radiographic density	**Radiographic contrast**
kV	increase	increased (darker)	low contrast (more shades of grey)
	decrease	decreased (lighter)	high contrast (fewer shades of grey)
mA	increase	increased (darker)	no effect
	decrease	decreased (lighter)	no effect
exposure time	increase	increased (darker)	no effect
	decrease	decreased (lighter)	no effect

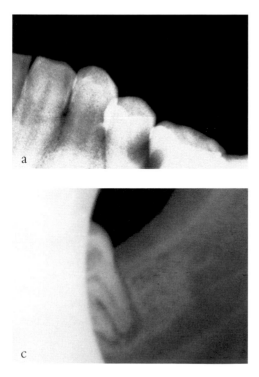

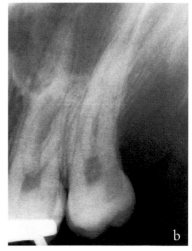

Fig 2-11 Common technique faults affecting intraoral radiography; a) incorrect film placement; (b) bending of the film; (c) incorrect alignment of the x-ray beam, causing "coning off".

25

Such a design is shown in Fig 2-12. Use of such devices has been shown to reduce reject rates in intraoral radiography and should be seen as essential for 21st century dental imaging. While these film holders were originally designed with film in mind, most manufacturers of digital equipment provide "sensor-holding" or "phosphor-plate-holding" devices that are comparable in design or compatible with the extraoral component of existing film holders.

For endodontic purposes, where a file is in the tooth for working length estimation, modified bite blocks that permit the patient to bite down correctly are available (Fig 2-13).

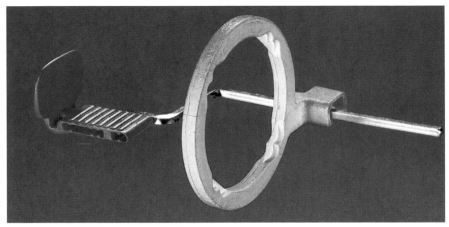

Fig 2-12 Modern film-holding/beam-aiming device used for periapical radiography. Note the extraoral aiming device.

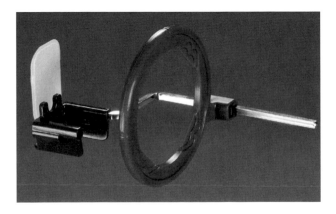

Fig 2-13 Film holder for endodontic use. The bite block is modified to permit a patient to bite upon it with an endodontic file in place.

Key Points

- The following features of a modern dental x-ray unit contribute to dose reduction:
  - high kV (60–70 kV)
  - constant potential
  - aluminium filtration
  - long open-ended position indicating devices
  - rectangular collimation.
- A small effective focal spot will improve image sharpness.
- The use of high kV machines and constant-potential units reduces radiographic contrast.
- The use of devices to hold the image receptor and to help align the x-ray beam is essential for optimal quality.

Further Reading

Environmental Health Directorate Health Protection Branch (Canada). Radiation Protection in Dentistry. Recommended Safety Procedures for the Use of Dental X-Ray Equipment. Safety Code 30. Environmental Health Directorate (Canada). 2000.

European Commission. Radiation Protection 136. European Guidelines on Radiation Protection in Dental Radiology. The safe use of radiographs in dental practice. EC, 2004.

Langland OE, Langlais RP and Preece JW. Principles of Dental Imaging. 2nd edn. Baltimore: Lippincott, Williams & Wilkins, 2002.

National Council on Radiation Protection and Measurements. Radiation Protection in Dentistry. NCRP Report No. 145. Bethesda, MD: NCRP, 2004.

National Radiological Protection Board. Guidance Notes for Dental Practitioners on the Safe Use of X-Ray Equipment. NRPB. London: Department of Health, 2001.

Whaites E. Essentials of Dental Radiography and Radiology. 4th edn. Edinburgh: Churchill Livingstone, 2006.

Chapter 3
Panoramic Equipment and Imaging

Aim

The aim of this chapter is to describe modern panoramic x-ray equipment, in particular those design features that improve safety and image quality.

Outcome

After reading this chapter the reader should be able to:
- give the indications for panoramic imaging
- list the functions of components of a panoramic machine
- outline how a panoramic image is formed
- describe how to position a patient correctly in a typical machine
- assess image quality
- identify common anatomical structures
- outline the additional features and programmes that are found on modern panoramic units.

Indications for Panoramic Imaging

The panoramic radiograph has several advantages over intraoral imaging. It is quicker and easier to perform than a set of full-mouth periapical views, and because all teeth and supporting structures are shown on one film it has an ancillary use for patient education.

There used to be a dose advantage in using a panoramic view over a set of full-mouth periapical views. However, using modern intraoral equipment and techniques this may no longer be the case. In addition, the resolution of the panoramic image is lower than obtained by intraoral imaging. The indications for panoramic imaging are limited to those situations where intraoral imaging is not practicable or realistic. This makes it ideally suited to the evaluation of large intrabony lesions, impacted third molars, the assessment of bony trauma and assessment of the bony parts of the temporomandibular joints.

In the general practice setting, panoramic radiography should not be used as a screening tool for new patients, as the prevalence of significant asymptomatic disease is low. The following indications for panoramic imaging are taken from *Selection Criteria for Dental Radiography*, a document published by the Faculty of General Dental Practitioners (UK):

• Where a bony lesion or unerupted tooth cannot be demonstrated on intra-oral radiographs.
• In a patient with a neglected dentition where clinically there are multiple carious teeth and there is concurrent generalised advanced periodontal disease.
• As part of an orthodontic assessment where there is a clinical need to know the state of the dentition and the presence or absence of teeth. (In addition, the British Orthodontic Society has produced guidelines on the use of radiographs in orthodontics.)
• In the assessment of third molars prior to surgical extraction.

Equipment

A typical panoramic machine and its components are shown in Fig 3-1.

• *X-ray tube head*. Produces the x-ray beam. The beam is aimed slightly upwards, towards the slot in the cassette holder.
• *Diaphragm*. The x-ray beam is collimated by the diaphragm to form a vertical slit-shaped beam. The x-ray beam width should be no greater than 5 mm.
• *Cassette holder*. Has a metal sheet at the front that prevents scattered x-ray photons reaching the cassette, which would otherwise degrade the image. There is a narrow vertical slot in the holder directly opposite the x-ray source. This ensures that only a small amount of the film is exposed at one time.
• *Cassette carriage*. Moves the cassette behind the cassette holder during the exposure.
• *Bite block*. Used to locate both upper and lower incisor teeth in an edge-to-edge relationship in the focal layer. It also separates the upper and lower teeth to prevent overlap.
• *Light-beam markers*. Used to position the patient correctly, to ensure that the teeth fall in the focal layer.
• *Head-holding apparatus*. Allows the patient's head to be immobilised once accurately positioned.
• *Handles*. Minimise movement of the patient.

Image Formation

Simultaneous rotational movements of the x ray source, cassette and cassette-holder in the horizontal plane produce a U-shaped focal layer of the

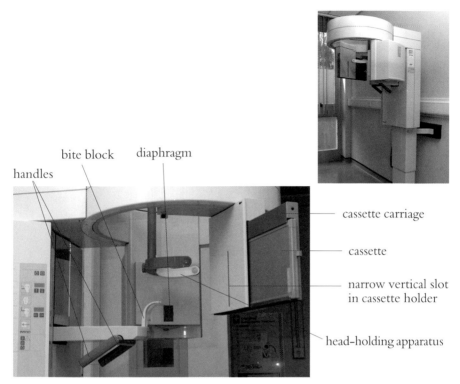

bite block   diaphragm

handles

cassette carriage

cassette

narrow vertical slot
in cassette holder

head–holding apparatus

Fig 3-1 An example of a panoramic machine, with the main components labelled.

teeth and jaws. During the exposure, the x-ray beam moves behind the patient, the cassette holder moves in front of the patient, and the cassette carriage and cassette move behind the slot in the cassette holder. These movements are shown in Fig 3-2.

The x-ray beam passes through the structures in the focal layer at the same speed as the cassette passes behind the slot in the cassette holder, ensuring those structures are sharply defined. The focal layer reflects the shape of the jaws in an "average patient", but it varies in shape depending on manufacturer. The thickness of the layer also varies; being narrower anteriorly than it is posteriorly. Some units use a continuously moving centre of rotation to produce the U-shaped focal layer (Fig 3-3). It should also be appreciated that the focal layer is three dimensional, with the height of the layer being determined by the height of the slit-shaped beam.

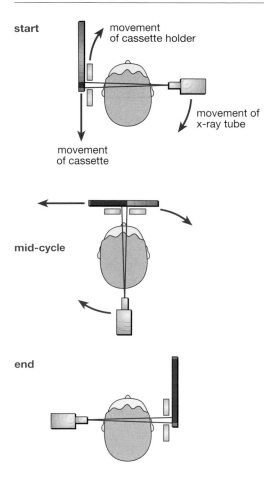

start

movement
of cassette holder

movement of
x-ray tube

movement
of cassette

mid-cycle

end

Fig 3-2 Diagram showing the movements of the x-ray tube, cassette holder and cassette during a panoramic exposure. (Based on a diagram provided by Mr E Whaites).

The image is magnified by between 10 and 30%. Magnification in the vertical and horizontal planes is equal only for those structures that fall into the centre of the focal layer. Therefore, uniform magnification of the teeth is seen only when the patient is positioned correctly and the shape of the jaws conforms exactly to the shape of the focal layer. Those structures outside the focal layer are distorted, blurred and often unrecognisable. Those structures that fall between the focal layer and the cassette tend to be narrowed in the horizontal plane and those structures located lingually are magnified in the horizontal plane. Distortion in the vertical plane is not generally as marked as in the

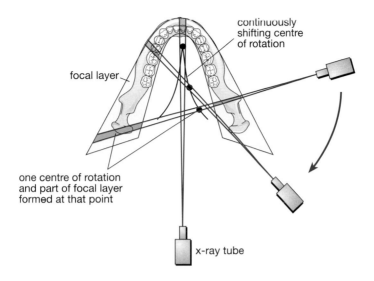

continuously
shifting centre
of rotation

focal layer

one centre of rotation
and part of focal layer
formed at that point

x-ray tube

Fig 3-3 Some machines use a continuously moving centre of rotation to produce the curved focal layer similar in shape to the "average jaws". This diagram shows three stages in this movement, the position of the x-ray tube and direction of the x-ray beam at these times, and the part of the image formed at these stages.

horizontal plane. Some studies have shown that there can be a narrowing of the focal layer if it is captured digitally, making patient positioning even more important.

The image is built up sequentially as the apparatus rotates about the patient, with an exposure time of 12–20 seconds for an adult. It is vitally important that the patient remains motionless during the exposure, to prevent movement artefacts on the image.

Procedure

Before the Exposure
- Confirm the identity of the patient.
- Ask the patient to remove dentures, removable orthodontic appliances, tongue studs, earrings, necklaces, glasses and hair ornaments which may be in the path of the x-ray beam.
- Set a suitable programme and exposure factors.

- Place a plastic sleeve on the bite block for control of cross-infection purposes.
- Position and instruct the patient correctly (Fig 3-4 and Table 3-1).

During Exposure
- Watch the patient during the exposure and check that they remain still.
- If the movement fails or the machine catches on the patient's shoulders and stops rotating, the exposure should be terminated to avoid localised high exposure of the patient.

After the Exposure
- The plastic sleeve is removed and discarded.
- The equipment should be wiped down using a suitable disinfectant wipe, ready for the next patient.
- The cassette is removed and the film processed.

Evaluation of the Image

Quality Assessment of the Panoramic Image
- The film should be clearly marked for right and left sides and must have legible patient identification. (Some machines have a name marker so that the film is marked prior to processing, helping to eliminate labelling errors).
- There should be no patient preparation errors, i.e. failure to remove dentures or other removable metallic objects will result in radiopaque shadows on the image.
- The patient should be correctly positioned so that the teeth and supporting bone fall within the focal layer and are clearly shown (Table 3-1).

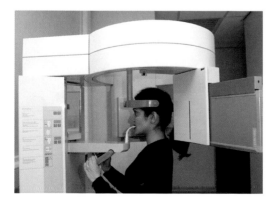

Fig 3-4 Patient positioned correctly for a dental panoramic radiograph.

Table 3-1 **The technique and importance of correct positioning of the patient for panoramic imaging**

Positioning the patient	Effect on image
Make sure the patient is standing or seated with the spine straight	Ensures only a faint ghost shadow of the cervical spine is visible in the anterior region
Instruct the patient to bite into the grooves on the bite block so the upper and lower incisor teeth are positioned edge to edge	Helps ensure both the maxillary and mandibular anterior teeth lie within the focal layer
Using the positioning lights, check that the median sagittal plane is vertical with no rotation of the head	Ensures that the molar teeth are of equal horizontal magnification and that only faint ghost shadows of the mandible are produced
Make certain that the Frankfort plane is horizontal, using the positioning lights	Ensures that the hard palate is projected above the apices of the maxillary teeth. The occlusal plane will then have a gentle curve with no/minimal overlap of the posterior teeth
There may be an additional vertical positioning light which should be positioned according to the manufacturer's instructions, often on the upper canine tooth	Helps to position the patient correctly antero-posteriorly so that the anterior teeth lie within the focal layer. The incisor teeth should be neither narrowed or widened
Immobilise the head using the head support	Reduces the chance of movement artefact. In some machines, the head support also sets the size of the focal layer
Ask the patient to close their lips around the bite block and press their tongue against the palate	Ensures no air shadows are seen superimposed on the anterior teeth and between the tongue and hard palate
Ask the patient to keep still and not to swallow during the exposure	Reduces the chance of movement artefacts and air shadows

- Exposure settings should have been chosen appropriate for the size of the patient. The image should be of sufficient density and contrast to distinguish enamel, dentine, pulp and the supporting bone.
- There should be no processing faults or errors due to faulty cassettes or screens.

A good quality panoramic image is shown in Fig 3-5a and 3-5b names the main anatomical features.

Normal Anatomy

The anatomical structures lying within the focal layer are seen clearly on the panoramic image (Fig 3-5). However, ghost shadows are also seen on the radiograph. These shadows are formed if the anatomical structure is located between the focus and the horizontal centre of rotation. Classically, ghost shadows are blurred, magnified and projected onto the opposite side of the film. They are more superiorly positioned than the real structure due to the slight upward angulation on the x-ray beam. The ghost shadows most commonly seen on a panoramic radiograph are shadows of the cervical spine, hard palate and mandible. These shadows are shown in Fig 3-6. Ghost shadows can make interpretation difficult as they can obscure the underlying real shadows.

Additional Programmes and Features on Panoramic Machines

Many panoramic machines now have additional programmes. The most common are described below.

Adjustable Focal Layer

Jaws vary in size, due mainly to the age, gender or race of the patient. Therefore, many machines allow a choice of focal layer size to allow for these differences. Additionally, some units have a choice of shapes for the focal layer to give even more flexibility. Unless the jaws fall within the focal layer there will be distortion of the image, so these features are potentially very valuable.

Field Limitation

Field limitation programmes permit selected areas of the jaws to be imaged. The simplest of these are the sectional panoramic programmes, which allow either the right or left side of the patient to be imaged. There are more sophisticated programmes that allow smaller, more specific areas of the jaw to be targeted. These may be used to investigate single teeth when periapical views are not possible.

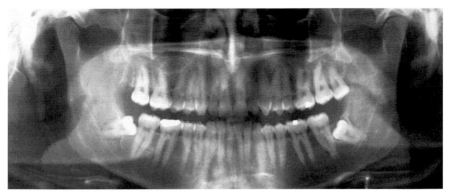

Fig 3-5 a) Good quality panoramic radiograph.

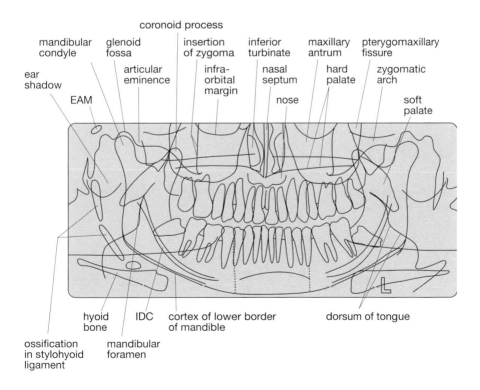

Fig 3-5 b) Diagram showing the main anatomical features seen on the radiograph. EAM = external auditory meatus; IDC = inferior dental canal.

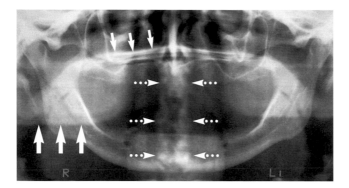

Fig 3-6 Panoramic radiograph of an edentulous patient showing the ghost shadows of the: cervical spine (small dotted arrows), hard palate (small solid arrows) and mandible (large solid arrows).

Most of the time, panoramic radiographs are taken to examine the teeth and supporting bone. Choosing a programme that only demonstrates the dentition can reduce the effective dose by 50%.

The vertical beam height should also be restricted to that required to expose only the area of clinical interest. These programmes can reduce exposure to the orbits and are incorporated into some "child mode" settings. In addition, these child mode programmes may automatically use a smaller or narrower U-shaped focal layer.

The European guidelines on radiation protection in dental radiology recommend the use of field limitation programmes as they are an easy and effective way of reducing dose.

A selection of images obtained using field limitation programmes is shown in Fig 3-7.

Cross-sectional Imaging
These programmes are used to obtain cross sections of the jaws. They are discussed in the chapter on implant imaging (Chapter 9).

Temporomandibular Joint Imaging
Most of the new panographic machines have a dedicated programme to radiograph the temporomandibular joints (TMJs). The majority of these views produce lateral views of the TMJs, although some can produce coronal slices as well. The lateral view commonly comprises an open and a closed view of

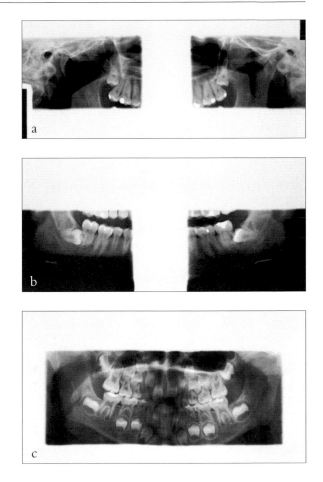

Fig 3-7 Some examples of images obtained using field limitation programmes;
a) posterior maxilla programme;
b) posterior mandible programme;
c) child programme (this particular setting automatically selects a smaller U-shaped focal layer).

each joint on the same film (Fig 3-8). For the closed view, the patient is positioned so that the teeth are in occlusion. This allows an assessment of condylar position within the mandibular fossa. The focal layer is often different to that of the standard panoramic programme, producing a cross-section that is more perpendicular to the condylar head, known as a "corrected lateral view". These views are useful in the imaging of bony disease of the joint, but they have limited use in general dental practice. This is because the majority of patients with TMJ problems have temporomandibular joint dysfunction syndrome – a condition with minimal radiographic changes.

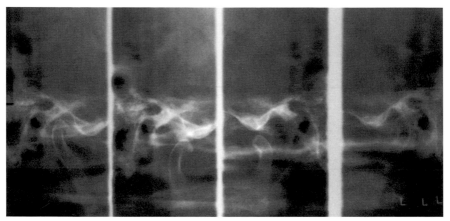

Fig 3-8 Example of an open and closed view of the left and right temporomandibular joints. Note the abnormal appearance of the right condyle.

Sinus Imaging

Some machines have a programme to produce a curved cross-sectional image through the maxillary antra (Fig 3-9). This view has applications in the evaluation of facial fractures because there is minimal superimposition from other bones over the area of interest. However, the use of this image is not widespread. It may also be used to investigate other conditions affecting the maxillary antra, such as cysts.

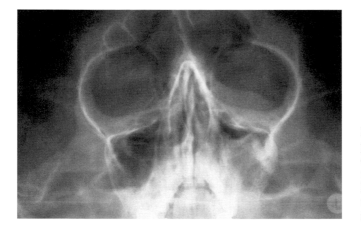

Fig 3-9 Midfacial panoramic radiograph showing the maxillary antra. Note the opacity in the base of the left maxillary antrum.

Exposure Settings
Modern panoramic machines are direct current (DC) units. As discussed earlier (Chapter 2), DC units produce an x-ray beam with a higher mean energy and deliver a lower skin dose to the patient than alternating current (AC) units. Another advantage is that there are no fluctuations in the energy of the x-ray beam, allowing an image of even density to be produced.

In older panoramic machines the ghost shadow of the cervical spine may substantially obscure the anterior region. Although the ghost shadow is an inherent shadow and cannot be eliminated completely, modern units have software to compensate for the ghost shadow by increasing the overall density in this area. This is achieved by increasing the exposure factors or by slowing down the rotation as the beam passes through the cervical spine.

Some digital panoramic machines boast automatic exposure control. This automatically adjusts the kV or mA to provide optimum penetration of the patient's tissues, producing an image with the correct overall density.

Cephalometric Attachments
Cephalometric radiology is often essential in the orthodontic assessment of a child patient. New panoramic machines can be purchased with a cephalometric attachment or they can be upgraded at a later time. The equipment comprises an arm that contains the head-positioning apparatus. This apparatus consists of ear posts which, when gently inserted into the external auditory meati, position the patient perpendicular to the x-ray source. The central ray of the beam is centred on the ear rods. The length of the arm ensures a long focus-to-film distance to keep magnification to a minimum. The recommended focus-to-film distance is 1.5–1.8 m. Constant magnification is produced, which may be as low as 10%. In addition, the head-holding apparatus may include a millimetre scale to allow accurate measurement of midline structures. Fig 3-10 shows a patient positioned for a lateral cephalometric radiograph.

A diaphragm is used to adjust the shape of the x-ray beam so that it is rectangular in shape. To visualise the soft tissue profile, a wedge filter is fitted at the tube head.

One of the disadvantages of these machines is the rectangular shape of the x-ray beam (Fig 3-11a). This means that the thyroid gland, cervical spine and skull vault are normally included in the field. If the thyroid is in the primary beam then lead shielding should be used because the gland is

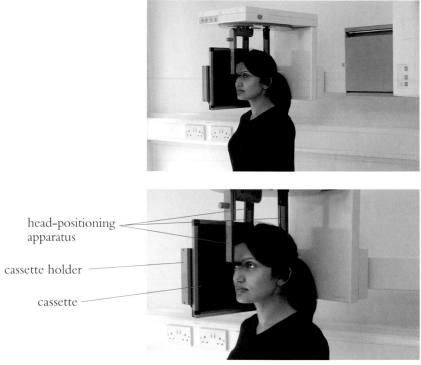

head-positioning
apparatus

cassette holder

cassette

Fig 3-10 Patient positioned for cephalometric imaging. The main components are labelled.

relatively radiosensitive. If, however, the beam is collimated to a triangular shape (Fig 3-11b), the dose can be reduced by 50% without losing any diagnostic information. It is recommended that all manufacturers should incorporate this feature into the design of cephalometric equipment, although at present it is not standard.

Key Points

- Image quality in panoramic imaging is inferior to intraoral imaging using packet film.
- The indications for panoramic imaging in general dental practice do not include "screening radiographs".

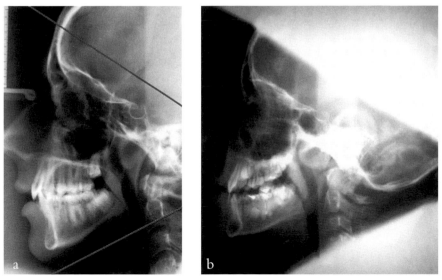

Fig 3-11 a) Good quality cephalometric radiograph. The teeth and important bony landmarks as well as the tissue profile can all be identified. Note that the beam is rectangular. If a triangular-shaped beam had been used (red lines), the dose would have been significantly reduced; b) cephalometric radiograph collimated in the recommended manner to exclude areas of no relevance to cephalometric analysis.

- Uniform magnification of the teeth is seen only when the patient is positioned correctly within the machine and the shape of the jaws conforms exactly to the shape of the focal layer.
- If panoramic imaging is indicated, suitable focal layer size, width and shape should be used along with appropriate field limitation whenever possible.
- Many panoramic machines can be purchased or upgraded to carry out cephalometric imaging.

Reference

Faculty of General Dental Practitioners (UK). Selection Criteria for Dental Radiography. 2nd edn. Eds: Pendlebury ME, Horner K and Eaton KA. Royal College of Surgeons of England, London, 2004.

Further Reading

European Commission. Radiation Protection 136. European Guidelines on Radiation Protection in Dental Radiology. The safe use of radiographs in dental practice. EC, 2004.

Langland OE, Langlais RP and Preece JW. Principles of Dental Imaging. 2nd edn. Baltimore: Lippincott, Williams & Wilkins, 2002.

National Radiological Protection Board. Guidance Notes for Dental Practitioners on the Safe Use of X-Ray Equipment. NRPB. London: Department of Health, 2001.

Chapter 4
Conventional Image Receptors

Aim

The aim of this chapter is to describe the modern choices available for the clinician using traditional image receptors for x-ray imaging.

Outcome

After completing this chapter, the reader should have an understanding of:
- the modern choices for non-digital capture of intraoral x-ray images
- the modern film/screen/cassette combinations available for extraoral radiography
- the modern choices for processing film-based images.

Intraoral Dental Film

While digital radiography is fast becoming the 21st-century option for dentists, it is likely that conventional film will remain the modality of choice for many dentists for economic reasons. By conventional film, we mean the direct x-ray sensitive film that is used for intraoral radiography. Only dentists use this type of film, with intensifying screen/film/cassette combinations used in all other types of conventional (non-digital) radiography. There are several reasons for this. Constructing tiny cassettes for use in the mouth is expensive and demanding. The challenge of cross-infection control means that disposable film packets are a convenience. It is, however, also important to remember that direct x-ray sensitive film offers a much higher resolution than do screen/film/cassette combinations (Fig 4-1).

Over the past century, there has been a steady pace of development in dental film technology, aimed principally at reducing the exposure necessary to produce the required "blackening" (optical density). The relationship between exposure and density is demonstrated by the film characteristic curve shown in Fig 4-2, which allows a simple visual method of relating a film's "speed" and "contrast". Films can be classified into groups, using capital letters as the group indicator. Until 1980 the fastest film commercially available was film of group D speed. This was superseded by E-speed film

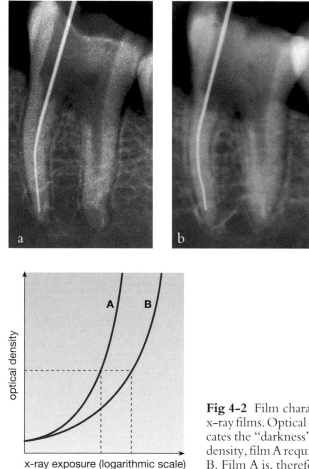

Fig 4-1 Two radiographs of the same tooth, taken a) using conventional, direct x-ray sensitive, intraoral film and b) using a screen/film/cassette combination. The intraoral film gives much better resolution, while the cassette film image shows some blurring in comparison.

Fig 4-2 Film characteristic curves for dental x-ray films. Optical density (vertical axis) indicates the "darkness" of the film. For the same density, film A requires less exposure than film B. Film A is, therefore, the faster film.

in 1981. This film could give the same density for about 50% of the exposure needed with D-speed film.

However, the E-speed film had a lower inherent contrast and greater sensitivity to aged and depleted processing solutions, which led to resistance to its adoption by many dentists. Furthermore, the very fact of it being "faster" meant that less than satisfactory darkroom safelighting might produce a significant fog level, which did not occur on the slower D-speed.

Subsequent developments in film technology produced improved E-speed emulsions and, most recently, films that fall into the F-speed group. Relative speed varies a little between manufacturers, but the change to F-speed film can allow 20–25% lower exposures than the same manufacturer's E-speed product.

The modern dentist who still uses conventional radiography should, therefore, use film speeds from the F-speed category. There is, however, an occasional barrier to this because the x-ray set cannot be easily adjusted to reduce exposures. As might be expected, this is particularly so for older machines. In such instances it is sensible to discuss the problem with your x-ray engineer and (in the UK) radiation protection adviser.

One final point worth mentioning is the use of "instant process" film. A number of manufacturers produce film that can be processed very quickly using a "monobath" solution, injected directly into the film packet. The films are, at best, D-speed, and image quality is invariably poorer than could be achieved with conventional processing. Therefore these should not be used for routine radiography. At best, their role would be in emergency situations, such as out-of-hours work when it is impracticable to organise normal processing, or during surgical procedures when a very rapid radiograph is needed.

Extraoral Radiography using Film Cassettes

Cassettes are used for panoramic, cephalometric and oblique lateral radiography. These are far more than simple rigid containers for a large film. Essentially, they include three different components:
• the outer casing
• a compressible layer
• the intensifying screens.

This arrangement is duplicated on either side of the hinged cassette shown in Fig 4-3 and is shown diagrammatically in Fig 4-4. The outer casing does, indeed, act as a container for the film and should be light-tight. A rigid cassette design is preferred as this is more robust and gives image quality advantages. Flexible cassettes, sometimes provided by manufacturers of panoramic x-ray equipment, are prone to light leaks (Fig 4-5) and poor film–screen contact (Fig 4-6).

The most important components in the cassette are the intensifying screens. These come in pairs; one is fixed to each side of the cassette. The film is

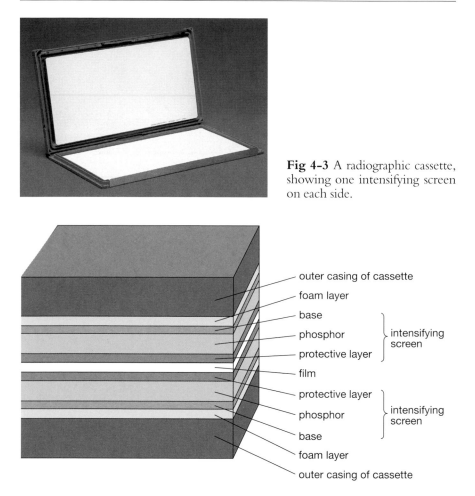

Fig 4-3 A radiographic cassette, showing one intensifying screen on each side.

Fig 4-4 A diagrammatic cross-section of a closed cassette containing a film. The film is sandwiched tightly between opposing screens.

placed between the screens. Intensifying screens work by absorbing the x-ray energy and converting it to light (fluorescence), which in turn exposes the film. Using intensifying screens rather than film alone allows x-ray exposures to be reduced enormously (by at least 90%).

The base material of the intensifying screens is a thin plastic layer, which supports the x-ray sensitive phosphor coat. It also helps in the imaging process

Fig 4-5 This poor-quality panoramic radiograph shows dense (black) artefacts along the upper edge of the film.
These are typical of light leakage into the cassette causing localised film fogging.

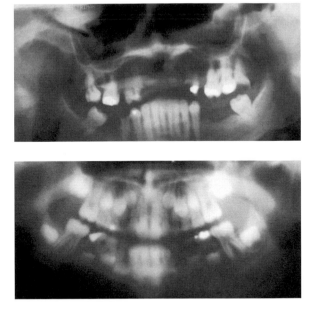

Fig 4-6 Poor film–screen contact results in considerable image unsharpness as light emissions from the screens diffuse before reaching the film.

by reflecting light from the phosphor on to the screens. In some cases this reflection is a property of the base material itself, and in others it is produced by a coating of titanium dioxide.

There are basically two types of screen: calcium tungstate and rare earth. The former has a long history, while the latter was first introduced in 1972. Calcium tungstate fluoresces at 440 nm (blue light). Many dental practices probably still use cassettes with this type of phosphor, but calcium tungstate absorbs x-rays and converts their energy to light very inefficiently. The alternative rare earth phosphors work far more efficiently. They vary in composition from manufacturer to manufacturer, but those used most frequently contain:

- gadolinium oxysulphide (terbium activated)
- lanthanum oxybromide (terbium activated)
- yttrium tantalite (niobium activated).

The first two of these emit light in the yellow/green end of the spectrum, while the third emits blue/ultraviolet light. Used properly, intensifying screens containing these materials absorb about 60% of the x-ray energy (compared with about 20% for calcium tungstate) and the efficiency of conversion to light is around 20% (compared with about 5% for calcium tungstate). This greater sensitivity and efficiency allows lower radiation doses to be used. Typically, there is a dose reduction of about 50%.

If you are not sure what type of screens you are using in your practice, it is fairly easy to find out. Take your cassette and open it so the screens are visible. Point a dental x-ray set directly at a screen and make an exposure while watching carefully. It is worth doing this with the room dark and with the x-ray set close to the screens as the emitted light is not bright. If you observe the screen you will see the colour of light emitted and can thus work out the screen type. One unfortunate problem is the blue/ultraviolet light emitted by the yttrium-containing rare earth screens. Nonetheless, the overwhelming majority of dental cassettes will follow the usual colour rules.

The film used must have a colour sensitivity matched to the emission colour of the screens. This is very important, because a mismatch will either give no image or, at best, a very faint image, which might cause the unwary to turn up the x-ray exposure.

In a modern dental practice, cassettes should be fitted with rare earth intensifying screens. The available screens come in different "speeds" (analogous to film speed), denoted by a number and a general rating, "high speed", "medium speed", etc. You should use the fastest film/screen combination consistent with satisfactory diagnostic results. European guidelines indicate that the speed should be at least 400 (high speed).

When selecting a film the choice may be between films with high contrast and films with wide latitude. As might be expected, the former produce very "black and white" images, while the latter give more grey tones (Fig 4-7). Despite the instinctive liking of many dentists for high contrast, research has shown that wide-latitude film is best for panoramic and cephalometric radiography as it reduces the prominence of areas of "burn-out". Such wide-latitude films are usually denoted by a suffix "L" to their manufacturer's name, for example T-Mat-L (Kodak) or HR-L (Fuji). While it is perfectly possible to mix film from one manufacturer with the screens from another, it is probably prudent to match them by manufacturer.

Processing of Film

Producing a radiograph that can be read requires that a film is processed properly. In order to explain what happens during processing, it is necessary to

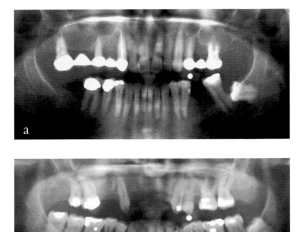

Fig 4-7 Panoramic radiographs produced on:
a) high-contrast and
b) wide-latitude film.
The high-contrast film produces more "burnt out" areas, while the wide-latitude film gives more even grey tones.

take one step back and consider first what happens when a film is exposed to x-rays.

The Latent Image

The emulsion of a film contains crystals of silver halide (largely bromide, with some iodide) in a supporting medium. These crystals contain very small traces of a sulphide impurity. On exposure, x-rays interact with bromide ions, stripping each of them of an electron. These free electrons gather around the sulphide impurity (sensitivity site) and "stick" there, making the region negatively charged. This attracts positively charged free silver ions, which are thus reduced to metallic silver. This collection of a few silver atoms in a crystal forms the "latent image". This is, of course, totally invisible to the eye and, in any case, is buried in the emulsion with all the unexposed silver halide crystals.

Development

Developer solutions contain reducing agents that convert silver halide crystals into metallic silver. The presence of the silver atoms in the exposed crystals, forming the latent image, means that the chemical reduction happens here first. As development continues, the latent image is enhanced to form large silver collections. Unexposed crystals, without a latent image, will not undergo this process unless development is continued for too long

51

or at excessively high temperatures. If this does occur, the result is fogging of the radiograph.

This chemical process is delayed at low temperatures and accelerated at high temperatures. Similarly, the process is less effective if the developer solution is too dilute or exhausted. The latter is usually a function of time, with three weeks being the usual limit for manual processing solutions.

Fixation, Washing and Drying

The fixer solution serves several purposes. It is acidic and halts development. The ammonium thiosulphate component of fixer removes unexposed crystals of silver halide, whereby the radiographic image becomes visible to the eye. Finally, it shrinks and hardens the emulsion.

A wash stage removes thiosulphate ions and salts. This is important because, if left, they would cause gradual discolouration of the film. Drying, of course, makes the emulsion stable and robust; it is easily damaged while wet. The stages of image formation and film processing are summarised in Fig 4-8.

Rapid Processing

Some manufacturers make rapid processing solutions, usually by increasing the concentration of chemicals. These can do the job of processing extremely quickly (15 seconds each for development and fixation) and so have uses in emergency situations or in cases where time saving is clinically helpful (e.g. endodontic working length estimation). However, in order to make such radiographs achieve archival quality it is important to place them back into fixer solution after clinical use. Otherwise, significant discolouration will occur over time.

Automatic Processing

Automatic processing has overtaken the manual method for most dentists, and it is probably essential kit for the 21st-century dental practice until the time is right for digital systems. Several manufacturers produce compact units suitable for processing intraoral and extraoral films (Fig 4-9).

Automatic processing reduces the time for processing, down to 4–6 minutes for delivery of a dry radiograph. Using higher temperatures than is customary for manual processing helps reduce the time, while the "squeezing effect" of the transport mechanism helps the exchange of solution in and out of the emulsion. The chemicals used are different from those used in manual methods, having been modified to cope with higher temperatures and shorter processing times. Therefore, it is important not to try using manual processing chemistry in automatic systems.

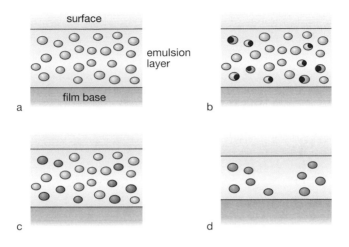

Fig 4-8 Diagrammatic representation of how a radiographic image is produced in the emulsion layer on a film surface; a) the unexposed emulsion contains crystals of silver halide; b) after exposure, specks of silver within crystals that were exposed to x-rays form a latent image; c) development of the film "grows" the latent image, converting the silver halide crystal to metallic silver; d) after fixation, the unexposed silver halide crystals are removed and the emulsion shrinks, leaving a visible radiographic image. Remember that on radiographic film the emulsion is on both sides of the film.

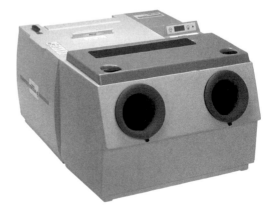

Fig 4-9 A typical modern automatic processing machine for dental radiography, including a daylight loading compartment. (Courtesy of Medivance Instruments Ltd).

53

Although automatic processing, when used properly, gives greater consistency in processing quality, it is fair to say that the final product quality is not quite so high as (optimally) manually processed film. This is related to a slightly higher fog level and graininess. In reality, however, most problems with automatically processed film reflect poor maintenance by the user, usually because equipment cleaning does not follow the manufacturer's protocol.

Adding to their utility, automatic processors often come with a daylight loading compartment, which avoids the need for a darkroom. In essence, however, this attachment is a very small darkroom itself. Fogging of films can arise either by placing the machine in or under bright light or by the loading compartment leaking light around its edge or through the arm holes. On large films, this manifests as fogging that gradually increases along the length of the radiograph (Fig 4-10).

Processing Quality Assurance
Consistent processing leads to consistent diagnostic quality. A low-contrast, pale film will reduce perception of dental caries and so has a very significant impact on patient care. Furthermore, if processing is suboptimal there is a risk of exposures being set higher than necessary to compensate. Consistency in processing is facilitated by carrying out a quality assurance programme. This encompasses a regular programme of duties, including:
- darkroom checks; cleaning, safelighting and light-tightness
- temperature and time checks in manual processing

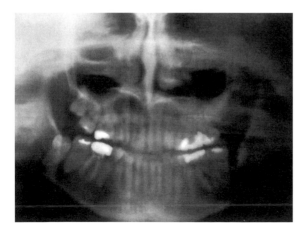

Fig 4-10 As your eyes move from your left to right across this radiograph, you may notice that the image gets darker and contrast gets worse. This is typical of fogging by light while the film was being fed into the automatic processor inside a daylight loading compartment. The right side of the image was last to enter the processor and thus suffered the greatest fogging.

- cleaning processing tanks
- maintenance of automatic processing equipment
- regular changes of chemistry
- processor monitoring.

The last of these, processor monitoring, is based on the use of standard test objects, which are radiographed to provide a "standard image". A reference image of this object can then be used as a standard, and regular test films can be compared with it. Obviously, as the standard object and exposure times are consistent, the only variable that might affect the quality of the image of the object is the processing.

The usual test object is some type of step wedge, often aluminium (Fig 4-11), which will provide an image that includes a range of grey tones. This is best for assessing contrast and overall density. Several manufacturers provide suitable test objects. However, to simplify the whole process, one manufacturer produces pre-exposed film strips for processor monitoring (Fig 4-12). A simple protocol of comparing test films against reference films is advised, with criteria for taking action if the test film densities deviate significantly from the reference image.

Viewing Radiographs on Film

Looking at a radiograph on film seems a simple task, but in fact your perception depends heavily upon the viewing conditions. A radiograph is merely a pattern of black and grey on a clear base. It is viewed by transmitted light. Thus, a lot depends upon the nature of the transmitted illumination. Too little or too much light reduces contrast and perception of detail.

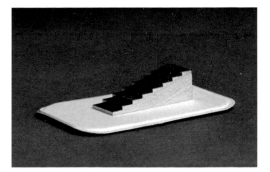

Fig 4-11 Small step wedge for processing quality control placed on a dental film packet. To be used for processor monitoring, the step wedge and film must be carefully exposed, using identical exposure factors, so that any changes in image quality on repeated radiographs can only be due to processing variation.

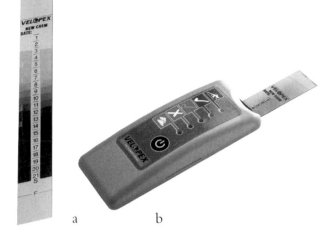

Fig 4-12 a) Pre-exposed film strip for simplified quality control of processing. Reference and test films could be read subjectively "by eye", but the manufacturer now produces an automatic reading device, b). (Courtesy of Medivance Instruments Ltd).

a   b

Of equal importance is the presence of "competing light". By this we mean light entering the viewer's eyes from around the film. For example, if you hold a radiograph up to a room light your eyes will receive all the light coming from around the film, reducing your perception of the radiograph itself. Thus, to obtain optimum information, radiographs should be placed on an illuminated viewing box and a mask used to block the extraneous light. Many "dental" viewing boxes are of a size suitable for panoramic radiographs so extra masking is not necessary, but for intraoral radiographs it is essential.

Unlike digital images, which can be magnified on the computer monitor, film radiographs are of a small size. Furthermore, there is more detail within an intraoral radiograph than can be perceived by the naked eye. Thus magnification is recommended (x2) for intraoral radiographs. This can be achieved easily by using a magnifying glass, but a combined magnifier/masking device is available (Fig 4-13), designed specifically for this purpose. Because there is less detail in panoramic and other extraoral radiographs, magnification is not essential, although it is still helpful when viewing a specific region of interest.

Summary

It is easy to be beguiled by the slick technology of digital imaging. It is worth remembering, however, that film (and film/screen/cassette combinations)

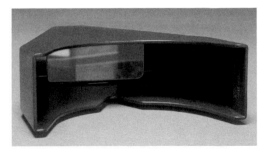

Fig 4-13 Commercially available combined magnifier/mask for viewing dental radiographs.

represents a tried and tested "low-tech" method of producing clinical images. It is relatively low cost and there is less risk of a system breakdown. If you are using conventional image receptors rather than digital radiography, what then can be considered "state-of-the-art" practice? The ideal recommendations are shown in Table 4-1.

Table 4-1 **"State-of-the-art" conventional film-based radiography**

Intraoral film		• Minimum E-speed; ideally F-speed
Film/screen/ casssette combinations	*Intensifying screens*	• Rare earth phospher
	Film	• Film matched to screen (most easily by using the same manufacturer's products • "Latitude" type film • Minimum speed of film/ screen combination of 400
	Cassette	• Rigid design
Processing		• Automatic processor • Maintenance programme • Quality assurance programme
Viewing conditions		• Dental light box • x2 magnification • Masking out of peripheral light

Further Reading

Carmichael F. The consistent image – how to improve the quality of dental radiographs: 2. The image receptor, processing and darkroom/film handling. Dent Update 2006;33:39–40,42.

White SC and Pharoah M. Oral Radiology. 5th edn. St. Louis: Mosby, 2005, Ch. 4, pp 68–82 and Ch. 6, pp 91–121.

Chapter 5
Digital Imaging

Aim

The aim of this chapter is to provide foundation knowledge for an understanding of digital x-ray imaging.

Outcome

At the end of this chapter, the reader should understand the differences between "analogue" and "digital", and the fundamentals of digital image data and how they can be manipulated.

Introduction

Digital is everywhere, from digital radio and television to digital cameras; the digital revolution is here. The word has become synonymous with quality, but what is "digital"? and why is it better than what we had?

Analogue

Before digital came along the world was exclusively analogue. Analogue refers to the continuous representation of a quantity. For example, if we measure the length of an object we can measure it in metres, centimetres, millimetres, micrometres, nanometres and so on. This applies to anything, for example size, colour and temperature. With analogue, wherever we measure and however finely we measure, there will always be something to see, continuously. This is illustrated in Fig 5-1, which shows a simple continuous analogue curve; we can look at any point on the curve and get an intensity value.

Digital

Whereas analogue is continuous, digital is discrete. That is, we represent a continuous signal by taking individual, discrete samples that together provide an approximation to the continuous signal. Fig 5-2 shows the same signal as in Fig 5-1, but now it has a grid overlaid to give the location of the sample points. Fig 5-3a shows the curve sampled at the closest points on the grid. The results give not only discrete positions but also discrete intensities. We can represent the curve digitally, that is numerically, as shown in Fig 5-3b.

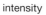

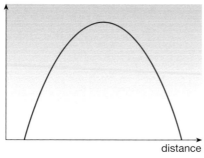

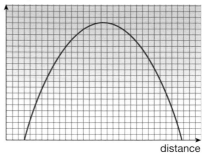

Fig 5-1 Analogue representation of a curve.

Fig 5-2 Discrete overlay grid used to sample the curve.

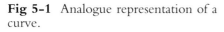

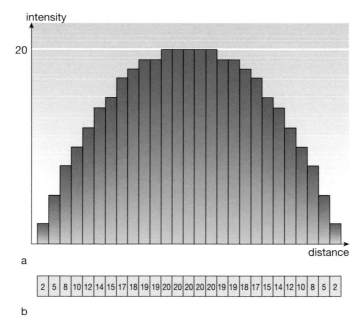

Fig 5-3 Sampled version of the curve; a) sampled at closest points; b) digital representation.

For an image we need a two-dimensional matrix, where each point has an image intensity value called a "greyscale". Each discrete point in an image is called a "pixel". The smaller the pixel size, the closer the digital sample is to the original signal (see Fig 5-4).

Advantages of Digital

The main advantage of digital radiography is that acquisition and display of images are separated. This means an image can be copied, stored remotely and viewed without limit. This has communication, workflow and archive advantages. The data can also be processed, using image processing, to preferentially enhance features of interest, which may arguably enhance diagnostic efficacy. Computer-aided diagnosis may also be possible, with the computer identifying features of interest and highlighting them for the user. All of these features add up to a faster and more efficient handling of diagnostic images. However, digital imaging is not without its limitations.

Disadvantages of Digital

The main technological limitation of digital imaging is the detector technology. The digital image will always be an approximation of the analogue signal, both spatially and in signal intensity. The better the digital detector, the closer we can get to the analogue presentation. Additionally, the patient dose for a digital system may need to be higher to achieve the same levels of noise as with film.

These are technology-related issues that may well be solved with technology advances. What cannot be improved is the loss of control of the image data. With film, the linked acquisition and display ensures consistent display and image probity. With digital, both of these factors can be varied at will and may have a significant impact on diagnostic quality. An example of this is where an image is compressed using "lossy" compression and transmitted electronically for remote viewing; the image data received by the viewer will contain compression artefacts. Additionally, the viewer may have a substandard monitor and so may not be able to see features originally identified.

These issues are not insurmountable but need to be considered for a digital diagnostic system, where loss of image quality may have serious consequences. An understanding of how the image data can be compromised is also important in order to maintain diagnostic quality.

Digital Image Parameters

Sampling Size

With digital data, there are several ways to describe the sampling size or sampling frequency of an image. These are:

* pixel size (mm or microns): the physical size of each pixel

- dots per inch (DPI): the number of dots (pixels) in a one-inch line
- line pairs per mm (lp/mm): the number of pairs of on/off pixels in 1 mm.

Of these, the term used most often in medical imaging is line pairs per mm. This measure has its roots in the term "cycles per mm", the analogue expression of frequency, and is the number of sine wave pairs in 1 mm. A sine wave is a continuous function and therefore cannot be used in digital imaging; it is replaced by the discrete line pairs per mm in digital images. For a 0.25 mm pixel size, the number of line pairs per mm is 2 (Fig 5-4). The equation that relates pixel size to line pairs per mm is:

$$lp/mm = \frac{1}{2 \cdot pixel\ size\ (mm)}$$

A comparison of line pairs per mm and the other measures is given in Table 5-1.

The highest frequency a digital image can display is called the "Nyquist frequency"; this is the point above which the digital system cannot represent the analogue signal. In the example shown in Fig 5-4, the highest frequency that can be represented is 2 lp/mm.

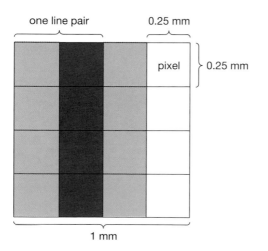

Fig 5-4 Example showing a group of pixels and a line pair. In this example, a pixel size of 0.25 mm and a spatial frequency of 2 lp/mm is shown.

Table 5-1 **Comparison of common expressions for digital resolution**

lp/mm	Pixel size (mm)	Pixel size (μm)	Approx. DPI
5	0.1	100	250
2	0.25	250	100
1	0.5	500	50

Bit Depth

Digital imaging requires computers. Unfortunately, computers do not work in decimal but in binary, and as a result they use "bits" and "bytes". As it is not possible to escape from this terminology it is worth clarifying what it means.

"Binary" is the number base 2, and therefore there are only two digits, 1 and 0. The value of each digit is determined by its order. Each digit is referred to as a "bit". There are four bits in a "nibble" and eight bits in a "byte". The number of bits available is referred to as the "bit depth". In a medical or dental image the bit depth is at least eight, which allows us to represent the values 0–255.

In order to find the number of decimal values, and so the number of levels of grey, allowed by a specific bit depth, raise 2 to the power n, where n is bit depth:

$$\text{Number grey levels} = 2^n$$

Table 5-2 shows the bit depths most commonly used in greyscale medical images and the number of levels of grey that each can reproduce. Fig 5-5

Table 5-2 **Commonly used bit depths for greyscale images**

Bit depth	Maximum decimal number (grey levels) that can be represented
8	256
10	1024
12	4096
16	65,536

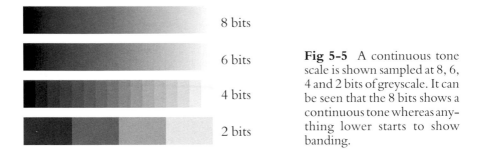

8 bits

6 bits

4 bits

2 bits

Fig 5-5 A continuous tone scale is shown sampled at 8, 6, 4 and 2 bits of greyscale. It can be seen that the 8 bits shows a continuous tone whereas anything lower starts to show banding.

illustrates the data loss that occurs if using less than eight bits. The higher the bit depth, the greater the number of grey levels and the closer we can represent the original analogue signal. However, increasing bit depth requires more space, as does increasing the matrix size (Table 5-3).

For these examples we are assuming greyscale images, the most commonly used in medical imaging; however, the same principles also apply to colour. With a 24-bit image, the bits are often divided into three colour groupings, or "channels": eight for red, eight for green, and eight for blue. Combinations of those bits are used to represent other colours. A 24-bit image therefore allows 16.7 million colours, or 256 levels of grey if each channel is set to be the same as the others.

Field Size
The pixel size is the size of the spatial sampling of an analogue signal. The number of samples therefore defines the area sampled. For example, ten 1-mm pixels will give a coverage of 10 mm², ten 0.1-mm pixels will cover only 1 mm², and for 10 mm² of coverage we would require 100 0.1-mm

Table 5-3 **Effect of increasing the image matrix on the image file size**

Image size (pixels)	Image size (kilobytes)
256 x 256	64
512 x 512	256
1024 x 1024	1024

pixels. This illustrates that both pixel size and number are required to determine the field size.

Impact on Image Presentation

Fig 5-6 shows an intraoral radiograph that can be described as having an image matrix of 641 x 452 pixels, 8 bits of greyscale (256 levels), with a pixel size of 0.064 mm. By zooming in on a region of interest it is possible to demonstrate how altering these parameters can materially affect the image quality and presentation.

Fig 5-7 shows how decreasing the available grey levels in the image results in a "banded image", which quickly loses clinical content. Fig 5-8 illustrates how making an image matrix smaller, with subsampling, but increasing the pixel size to retain the same physical size as the original produces a "pixelated" image.

If the image is subsampled but the pixel size is not changed (Fig 5-9), the image still "looks" correct, albeit smaller, but the same level of data loss will be achieved as in Fig 5-8.

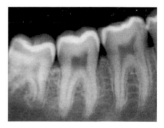

Fig 5-6 Example intraoral digital dental radiograph (8 bits greyscale, 641 x 452 pixels, 0.064 mm pixel size).

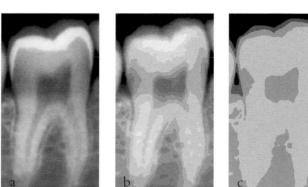

Fig 5-7 Effect of decreasing bit depth (shown magnified);
a) 8 bits, 256 grey levels;
b) 4 bits, 16 grey levels;
c) 2 bits, 4 grey levels.

65

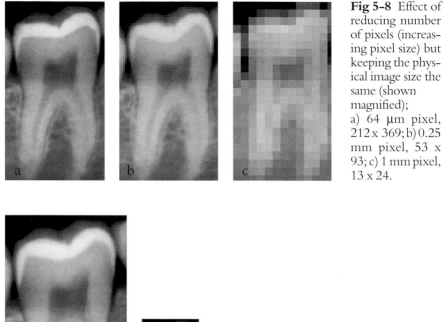

Fig 5-8 Effect of reducing number of pixels (increasing pixel size) but keeping the physical image size the same (shown magnified); a) 64 µm pixel, 212 x 369; b) 0.25 mm pixel, 53 x 93; c) 1 mm pixel, 13 x 24.

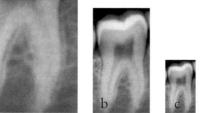

Fig 5-9 Effect of reducing number of pixels but keeping pixel size the same, i.e. image size decreases (shown magnified); a) 64 µm pixel, 212 x 369; b) image (a) at half size 106 x 185 pixels; c) image (a) quarter size 53 x 92 pixels.

Image Compression

Image compression is a method for reducing an image's size by mathematically analysing the image to allow it to be redefined in a smaller file size. The compressed image can then be reconstituted using the same algorithms to get back to the "original" image. There are two approaches to image compression, referred to as "lossless" and "lossy". These are exactly as they sound; lossless compression gives back exactly the same image, whereas lossy compression may lose some of the image content. In images such as photographs this may not be too high a cost in order to achieve a significant reduction in file size. However, for clinical images there is the issue of loss of diagnostically relevant information.

Generally, in medical imaging lossless compression is used, achieving a compression rate of approximately 2.2:1. There is conflicting evidence about the use of lossy compression. Some studies claim that 5:1 compression may be acceptable (see Further Reading), while others advise against the use of lossy compression. With the falling cost of data storage and the increasing speeds of networks, file size will be less of a concern to many users, in which case lossless compression should be used. For large institutions, or where storage space is an issue, it is suggested that lossy compression be used with caution, and only after the clinical risk has been considered for each examination type. One of the simplest forms of lossless image compression, and which clearly demonstrates the process, is run–length encoding.

Run–length Encoding
Run–length encoding is one the earliest and simplest methods of image compression. It works by running sequentially through the image counting the number of consecutive pixels with the same value. A new data file is then created using only the count and intensity values. This new data file will not be recognisable as an image, but it can be decoded by using the opposite process.

For example, consider a small 7 x 7 image matrix. This is represented in its original form by 49 data points (Table 5-4a). Using run–length encoding, the amount of data can be effectively halved (Table 5-4b).

Table 5-4a **Simple image matrix with 49 data points**

1	1	1	1	3	3	3
3	3	3	3	4	4	5
5	6	5	4	2	2	2
7	7	7	4	4	4	4
5	5	5	5	5	5	5
5	5	5	5	5	5	5
1	1	1	2	2	2	2

Table 5-4b **Compressed image matrix.** (The blue figure indicates the count and the black number the intensity. The file size is now only 26 data points: a 1.88:1 compression rate).

4	1	7	3	2	4	2
5	1	6	1	5	1	4
3	2	3	7	4	4	14
5	3	1	4	2		

This type of encoding works extremely well where there are large areas of homogenous intensity, such as the background and collimators on radiographic images. For images that change often, little or no compression may be achieved. Therefore, more complex algorithms are required for effective compression. One that is commonly used is the lossy algorithm called JPEG compression. There is, however, a newer version of JPEG called JPEG2000, which has a true lossless mode and so is suitable for medical images.

JPEG2000 Compression
JPEG2000 is the latest generation in the JPEG image compression family. It replaces the original discrete cosine transform with a set of algorithms called "wavelets". JPEG2000 is of particular interest as it was added to the DICOM standard (see Chapter 8) in 2001 and can routinely achieve lossless compressions of between 2:1 and 3:1. The method of operation is too complex for discussion here and the reader is referred to the text of Gonzalez and Woods (see Further Reading). It can, however, be used to demonstrate the potential impact of compression on image quality.

Fig 5-10 shows an intraoral image compressed using lossy and lossless modes of JPEG2000. To illustrate image degradation, difference images (showing the difference between the original and the compressed images) are also shown. The maximum lossless compression ratio is 7:1. At 10:1 there is a loss of high-frequency data across the image, at 100:1 image structures are beginning to be lost, and at 1000:1 the image is clearly non-diagnostic. This example indicates the potential of image processing for compression of image data. However, image processing can also be used to enhance the presentation of the image.

Image Processing

As stated previously, one of the advantages of digital images is that they can be processed to order to modify the presentation of the image. This is done either for consistency of presentation, for example to make digital images look more film-like, or to enhance or suppress an image feature to aid diagnosis.

All digital images are processed; a raw image has a wide latitude and, therefore, low contrast. In addition, image artefacts inherent in the acquisition of the image may be removed. These artefacts are typically dead pixels, system noise, scan lines or non-homogenous backgrounds. Usually, the clinical user will not be aware that the image is processed, and if the image presentation is satisfactory no further processing will be required. However, most image viewing software allows the user a modest amount of image processing to

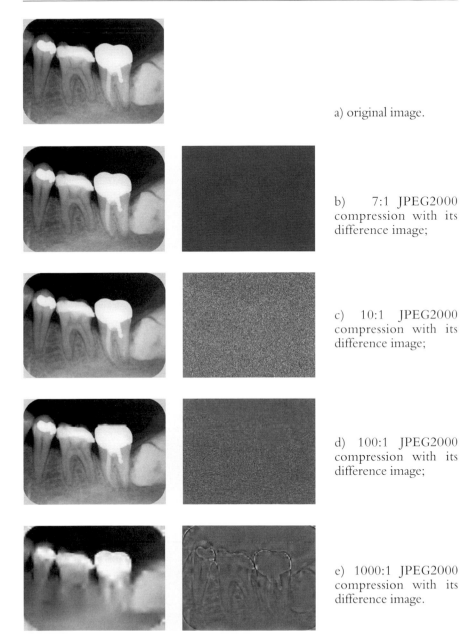

a) original image.

b)   7:1 JPEG2000 compression with its difference image;

c)   10:1 JPEG2000 compression with its difference image;

d)   100:1 JPEG2000 compression with its difference image;

e) 1000:1 JPEG2000 compression with its difference image.

Fig 5-10 Increasing the level of JPEG2000 compression results in lossy compression above a ratio of 7:1 for this image. The loss of clinical information becomes more evident as the ratio increases.

enable them to "tweak" the image. This processing usually falls into two categories: lookup table (LUT) adjustment and convolution processing.

Lookup Tables

Digital images are two-dimensional matrices with a third dimension relating to the intensity of each pixel. When displaying the image it is possible to alter the presentation of the data through a LUT. This maps the input intensity through a function to the output intensity, which alters the perceived brightness and contrast in the image. This process does not have to be permanent; a good example is the contrast and brightness functions of image viewing software.

It is useful to describe an LUT graphically, by plotting the input x against the output y. For a perfect reproduction of the input, the graph would show a straight line with a gradient of 45° (Fig 5-11). To alter the contrast of the output, the gradient of the line is altered (Figs 5-12 and 5-13), and to alter the brightness the line is shifted in the x direction (Figs 5-14 and 5-15). Using a non-linear curve allows for the image content in a certain intensity range to be preferentially enhanced or suppressed.

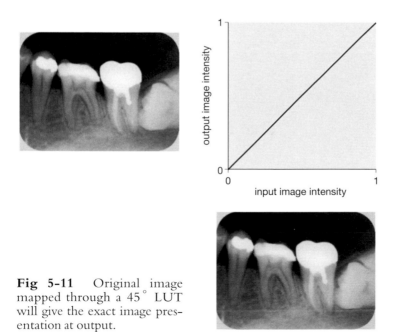

Fig 5-11 Original image mapped through a 45° LUT will give the exact image presentation at output.

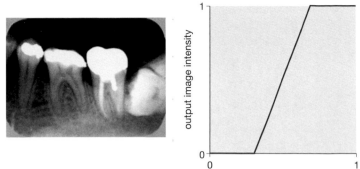

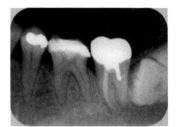

Fig 5-12 Original image mapped through an increased gradient LUT will give a high contrast image. Note that all levels in the top one-quarter of the input range will be mapped to white at the output, and grey levels in the bottom one-quarter of the range will map to black at the output.

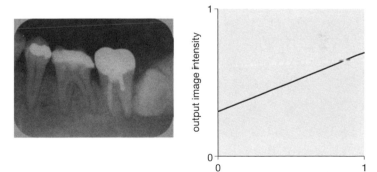

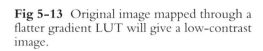

Fig 5-13 Original image mapped through a flatter gradient LUT will give a low-contrast image.

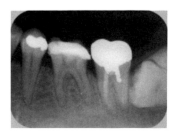

71

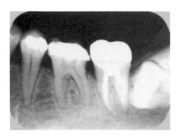

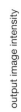

Fig 5-14 Original image mapped through a LUT shifted to the left will produce a bright image; again, all input levels in the top one-quarter of the input range will be mapped to white. Black at the input will be mapped to mid-grey at the output.

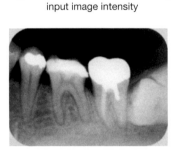

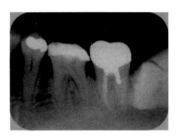

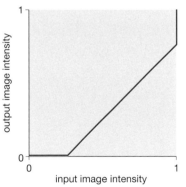

Fig 5-15 Original image mapped through a LUT shifted to the right will conversely produce a dark image.

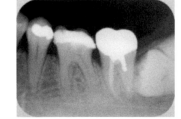

Simple Convolution Filtering

There is a vast array of complex algorithms that can be applied to a digital image. Even the novice user of a dental digital radiography system will be familiar with a number of simple image processing tools, yet they are unlikely to be unaware of what "clicking the mouse" actually achieves.

The convolution filter is a simple yet powerful image processing tool often used in medical applications and is a good introduction to image processing. It works by convolving the image matrix with a filter matrix called a "kernel". The kernel is applied sequentially to the image, and the result of the convolution is written back to the image at the point of the central element of the kernel or to a new image to preserve the original data. There is no limit to the kernel size, and even a 3 x 3 kernel size can have a dramatic impact on the image. However, in medical imaging we are usually trying to enhance the image without introducing image processing artefacts that may distract the viewer or mimic pathology.

Convolution filtering can be illustrated with a simple blurring kernel, as follows.

The kernel is applied to a region of the image, usually the top corner (in dark shading), which is the same size as the kernel.

($\otimes$ = convolution process)

The image segment is then convolved with the kernel.
For the shaded region:

$$(1 \times 1) + (2 \times 1) + (3 \times 1)$$
$$+ (1 \times 1) + (2 \times 1) + (3 \times 1)$$
$$+ (1 \times 1) + (2 \times 1) + (3 \times 1) \quad = 18/9 = 2$$

This result is then normalised to the sum of the kernel to ensure the intensity of the image is preserved. For this region = 18/9 = 2. This new pixel value is then written to the centre of the region or a new image.

This process is then repeated by moving the kernel sequentially over the image:

until the whole image is processed.

In this example we can see that the edge, with a peak intensity of 3 in the image has now been reduced to 2.3 in the final image. The result is that the new image is a blurred version of the original (Fig 5-16).

The kernel actually used on the image in Fig 5-16 was a 63 x 63 blur filter as a 3 x 3 blur filter would not be easily seen. This illustrates that the blur filter

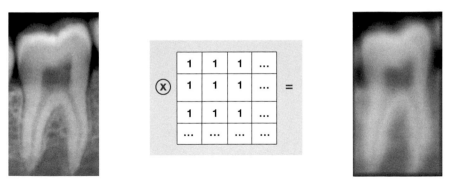

Fig 5-16 Effect of a simple blurring kernel form of image processing. The original image is on the left and the final image is on the right.

is effectively a frequency filter, with a small size blurring out only the very small or high-frequency features and a large filter blurring the larger, low-frequency features. Also note the banding around the edges of the processed image as a region half the kernel size minus 1 at the edges cannot be processed.

Other examples of simple processing are given in Figs 5-17 and 5-18. It should be noted that unlimited permutations of processing can be applied. One that has been widely adopted in medical imaging is unsharp mask subtraction (UMS), which employs convolution filtering with image arithmetic.

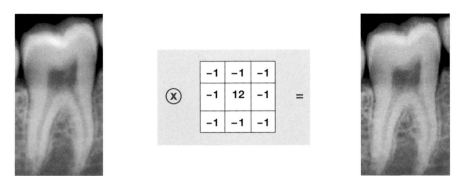

Fig 5-17 Effect of a low level sharpen filter. The original image is on the left and the final image is on the right.

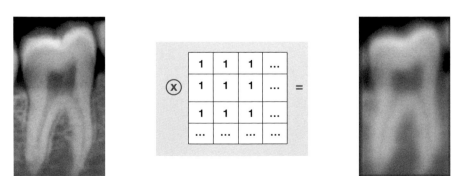

Fig 5-18 Effect of a pixel shift filter. The original image is on the left and the final image is on the right.

Unsharp Mask Subtraction

UMS in its simplest form requires the source image to be blurred using a very large kernel to leave only the low-frequency content in the image (Fig 5-19a). This is then subtracted from the original, the result being the high-frequency information, such as edges (Fig 5-19b). A percentage of this is then added back onto the original image to produce the final result (Fig 5-19c).

Although a very simple process, a great deal of control over the look of the final image can be achieved by altering the blur kernel size and the amount of the high-frequency image added back onto the original. This algorithm

Fig 5-19 a) Unsharp mask subtraction; blur stage. The original image is on the left and the blurred image on the right.

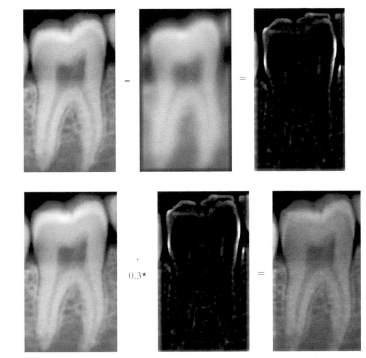

Fig 5-19 b) Unsharp mask subtraction, subtract stage; the image on the left is the original, the middle is the blurred image and the image on the right is high-frequency.
c) addition stage; the image on the left is the original, the middle is high-frequency and the image on the right is UMS.

has been used by many manufacturers to enhance medical images. The result can be seen to have improved contrast and high-frequency enhancement. It is important to note that this process can introduce an edge band around high-intensity boundaries, which may in some conditions mimic pathology. For further reading on image processing the text of Gonzalez and Woods is highly recommended.

Further Reading

Fidler A, Likar B, Skaleric U. Lossy JPEG compression: easy to compress, hard to compare. Dento Maxillo Facial Radiology 2006;35(2):67–73.

Gonzalez RC, Woods RE. Digital Image Processing. 2nd edn. Upper Saddle River, N.J.: Prentice Hall, 2002.

Ringl H, Schernthaner RE, Bankier AA, et al. JPEG2000 compression of thin-section CT images of the lung: effect of compression ratio on image quality. Radiology 2006;240(3):869–77.

Chapter 6
Direct Digital Imaging

Aim

The aim of this chapter is to provide a comprehensive understanding of direct digital x-ray imaging in dentistry.

Outcome

After reading this chapter the reader should be able to:
• understand the technology underlying direct digital imaging
• identify the differences between it and conventional film radiography
• see the clinical implications of using direct digital sensors.

What is Direct Digital Radiography?

Direct digital radiography involves the acquisition of digital data *without* an intermediate stage between exposure and image production. This is in contrast to indirect digital radiography (see Chapter 7), which requires an intermediate stage between the exposure of the patient and obtaining the image (i.e. the reading of a phosphor plate).

Direct digital imaging is achieved using a solid-state sensor to detect x-rays. All sensors have the same basic design, with a detection stage and a readout stage, although there are differences between sensors according to manufacturer and their clinical use (intraoral, panoramic or cephalometric radiography).

X-ray Detection

There is a vast array of dental x-ray equipment on the market that uses direct digital technology. Abbreviations such as CCD and CMOS are freely used in manufacturers' literature. In this section we hope to cast some light on this highly technical subject.

In direct digital imaging, the detection of x-rays may be through either *direct* or *indirect* conversion. This is not to be confused with direct or indirect *detection* but relates to the *conversion* of the x-rays to an electronic signal. These methods are described in more detail later, but both rely on solid-state materials at some stage in the image production.

Solid-state Materials

All direct digital detectors are solid-state *devices*; this means that they have no moving or mechanical parts. The device is a solid object, usually comprising electronic circuitry such as diodes and transistors; a good example is computer memory. These components are made from solid-state *materials*; materials that have properties that can be exploited at the material level, such as being semiconducting or superconducting. Many solid-state materials are crystalline, although amorphous materials (those with no ordered structure) are used in x-ray sensors. The two most commonly used are amorphous silicon (aSi) and amorphous selenium (aSe). These two materials are, however, usually used in completely different ways, with aSe being used for x-ray detection and aSi used for readout.

Indirect Conversion
At the time of writing, the most common technology for x-ray detection uses an indirect conversion method. The term "indirect" relates to the fact that the x-rays, incident on the detector, do not directly induce an electronic signal, but need to go though a secondary process. In this case, the process is the production of light by a scintillator.

X-ray scintillation is the conversion of x-ray photons to visible light photons. It is a well known property of some materials and has been used extensively in medical imaging, both in the phosphor plate in film screen cassettes and in the entrance phosphor on image intensifiers. Common materials used in digital detectors are the rare earth gadolinium oxysulfide (GdO_2S_2) and caesium iodide (CsI). GdO_2S_2 is used in its amorphous state (Fig 6-1a) as a light-emitting layer in the sensor sandwich.

CsI can also be used in this way, but newer methods can grow the columnar crystal of CsI directly onto the detector surface (Fig 6-1b). This has significant advantages: the detection layer can be thicker so that more light is produced than with GdO_2S_2, increasing the efficiency of the sensor; and it has less scatter than an amorphous material, as the crystal structure acts like a light pipe, resulting in theoretically greater detail resolution. Both emit green light that is detected by discrete photosensitive sites to be converted into an electric signal (Fig 6-2).

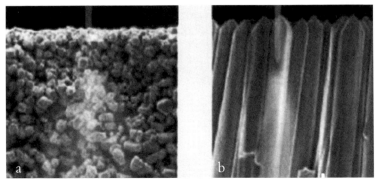

Fig 6-1 Electron microscope images of scintillators used in indirect conversion of x-rays; a) GdO₂S₂ amorphous structure; b) CsI columnar structure. The amorphous structure of the GdO₂S₂ and columnar structure of the CsI can be clearly seen. (Courtesy of Varian X-ray Products).

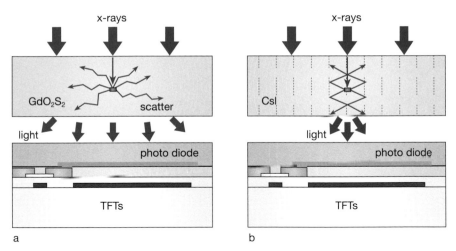

Fig 6-2 Examples of indirect conversions using a scintillator and a thin film transistor (TFT) array; a) GdO₂S₂ scintillator; b) columnar CsI scintillator.

Direct Conversion

With direct exposure sensors there is no scintillator. Instead, the x-rays are directly converted to a charge in the material through the photoelectric effect. This occurs in both aSi and aSe, although the conversion is not very efficient in the former. Currently, the material of choice for direct conversion is aSe.

81

X-ray exposure produces a charge (positive and negative) in the selenium, the size of which is proportional to the quantity of x-rays incident upon it. By placing a high voltage (kilovoltage) across the aSe, these charges can be moved to the surface to produce an electric current (Fig 6-3). This current is stored in a matrix of discrete capacitors that can then be read.

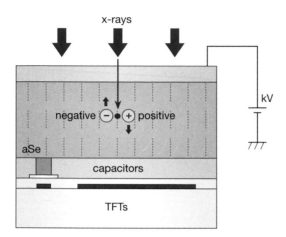

Fig 6-3 Example of direct conversion using an aSe detector: kV = kilovoltage.

Image Readout

In reading out the image data, three parameters need to be recorded: the pixel x position, the pixel y position and the signal intensity at that site. The x and y positions can be acquired either by direct addressing, as with a thin film transistor array (TFT), or by coupled readout, as used in charge-coupled devices (CCDs).

TFT

A thin film transistor (TFT) array is exactly as its name suggests: an array of up to millions of transistors made of silicon on a glass substrate. The transistors are used in conjunction with capacitor or photodiode elements to allow direct addressing of individual charge sites. TFTs can be used with either direct or indirect conversion devices. This technology is also used in liquid crystal displays (LCDs), where each individual transistor is used to control the state of the liquid crystal to allow light to be transmitted. The advantages of the TFT are the ability to address each of the individual transistors for direct readout and that physically large matrices, with many millions of transistors, can be made.

CCD

A charge-coupled device (CCD) is an image sensor consisting of an array of linked, or coupled, light-sensitive capacitors built on an aSi layer. CCDs are generally used with indirect conversion devices, and it is one of the most common technologies used for dental sensors. The image is read out sequentially by shifting an entire readout row of charges down into a readout buffer. When a row is moved into the readout buffer all the rows above are moved down as well. The row number gives the y coordinate. To obtain the x coordinate, the row is sampled by shifting each charge out of the readout buffer into the detection electronics, one element at a time (Fig 6-4).

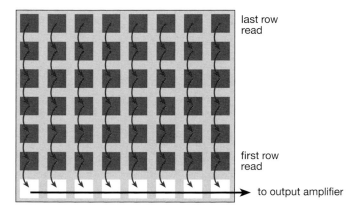

last row
read

first row
read

to output amplifier

Fig 6-4 Schematic of the readout process of a CCD sensor.

This is the same technology as used in digital cameras. One disadvantage of a CCD is that the sensor can only be made quite small, up to a maximum of about 4 cm, although it is possible to get around this limitation by joining detectors together. The advantages are that CCDs are relatively cheap and have a near 100% fill factor. A radiograph showing the construction of a CCD detector is shown in Fig 6-5.

CMOS

Complementary metal oxide semiconductor (CMOS) technology is commonly used in integrated circuit microchips, such as computer central processing units (CPUs) and memory chips. A CPU can contain over 10 million active elements. The production processes for these devices are well established, making production extremely cheap. This technology has been

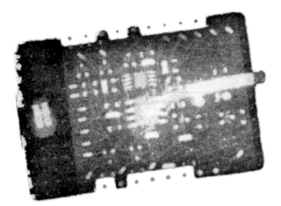

Fig 6-5 A radiograph of a direct digital CCD detector, showing the active area and readout electronics.

successfully employed for the construction of a light-detection device, in direct competition to the CCD, and also for direct conversion sensors. In the CMOS detector, each photodetector site also incorporates readout electronics (Fig 6-6).

The main disadvantage of the CMOS device is that it is less efficient than the CCD due to the lower fill factor (see below). A good comparison of the merits of CCD and CMOS technologies can be found in *CCD vs. CMOS* by Dave Litwiller (see Further Reading).

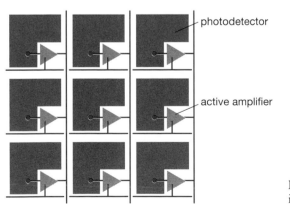

photodetector

active amplifier

Fig 6-6 CMOS sensor showing the "onboard" electronics.

Fill Factor

The fill factor relates to the area of the pixel site available to detect the light photons generated by the scintillator. In a CCD, all of the pixel area is available and as such a CCD has a 100% fill factor. The CMOS device, however, requires space on each pixel element for the "onboard" electronics. The more electronics present, the lower the fill factor. If 25% of the area were electronics, the device would have a 75% fill factor. One method used to compensate for lower fill factors is to use micro lenses to focus the available light to the active areas (Fig 6-7).

Pixel Binning

One method employed by sensor manufacturers to decrease sensor noise is to use pixel binning. This method works by sampling several pixels and averaging the result to produce a larger effective pixel. The reason this is used is that smaller sampling areas on the sensor result in lower photon detection, increasing the noise at the pixel. By sampling, for example, four

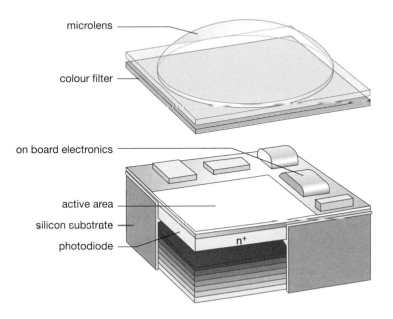

Fig 6-7 A CMOS pixel photosensor with a fill factor of about 60%, showing the micro lens used to focus the available light onto the active area.

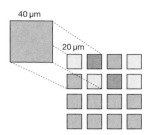

Fig 6-8 Pixel binning allows the noise in an image to be reduced by combining four pixels into a larger pixel. This reduces the resolution of the sensor but requires less radiation for the same noise level.

pixels at 20 x 20 µm into one pixel at 40 x 40 µm, the noise can be reduced (Fig 6-8). This is usually implemented by system designers as "standard" and "high-resolution" modes. The standard mode has larger pixels and requires less radiation than the high-resolution mode for the same noise level.

Electronics

Once the data have been read out from the sensor, a lot of processing is still required to generate a usable image (Fig 6-9). This includes digitisation of the signal amplitude, amplification and noise-reduction. These processes are too detailed for this text, but it is important to note that even if the same detector is used in two competing systems, as is often the case, bespoke electronics and signal processing components can result in significant differences in image quality between the two systems.

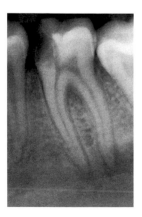

Fig 6-9 Intraoral radiograph produced using a CsI indirect conversion CCD sensor.

Comparisons with Film

It is inevitable when considering new technologies that comparisons are drawn with the existing technology. In the case of digital imaging the comparisons are, of course, with film. The comparisons are not only in terms of image quality but also dose and usability.

Image Quality
Digital imaging is a technology-limited process and so as advances are made in technology the image quality will improve. A current typical specification for one manufacturer's intraoral size 2 detector is shown in Table 6-1. There have been academic publications on the subjective quality of the competing technologies (see Further Reading), and there seems to be little doubt that current direct digital sensors are diagnostically suitable for dental applications.

Table 6-1 **Comparison of size 2 film with a direct digital size 2 sensor from one manufacturer.** (The pixel binning is used for the standard mode. This sensor is particularly thin; several other manufacturers' products exceed 5 mm in thickness)

Device	External dimensions (mm)	Thickness (mm)	Active area (mm)	Limiting resolution (lp/mm)
Film size 2	41 x 31	<1	41 x 31	>20
Direct digital size 2 High resolution	43 x 32	3.2	36 x 26	>22
Direct digital size 2 Standard resolution	43 x 32	3.2	36 x 26	>12

There are quantitative measures that allow us to compare the image quality of competing systems, the most comprehensive of which is the detective quantum efficiency (DQE). This is quite a complex measurement, but it allows the entire performance of a system to be compared with another. The DQE is expressed as a percentage, where 100% is a perfect system. Fig 6-10 shows the DQE curves for an indirect capture CCD intraoral detector and E-speed film. It can be seen that at the low frequencies, i.e. the physically large components in an image, the DQE of the digital device is about three times that of film. However, as the frequency increases, the poorer

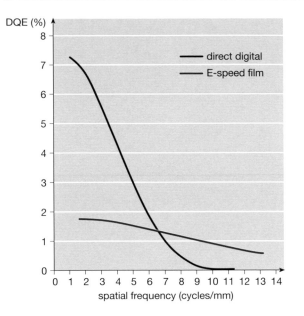

Fig 6-10 DQEs for E-speed film and a CsI indirect capture CCD intraoral detector.

frequency response of the digital sensor causes its performance to drop off at around 10 lp/mm. The net effect is that this direct digital detector can deliver the same image quality as film for approximately half the dose. Alternatively, it can produce twice the image quality for the same dose, assuming the sensor is not saturated (for an explanation of this phenomenon see Fig 6-12).

Resolution
The resolution response of a system is comprehensively described by the modulation transfer function (MTF). An MTF of 1 indicates that a frequency in the image is transferred perfectly, while an MTF of 0 indicates that the frequency is not transferred at all. Because a digital system is sampled its limiting resolution is lower than that of film (see Chapter 5). This is seen when comparing the MTF of an indirect capture CCD intraoral detector with the MTF of E-speed film (Fig 6-11).

Dose Considerations
One major claim made by some manufacturers of dental digital radiography equipment is that a much lower radiation dose is achievable compared with conventional radiography. How true is this?

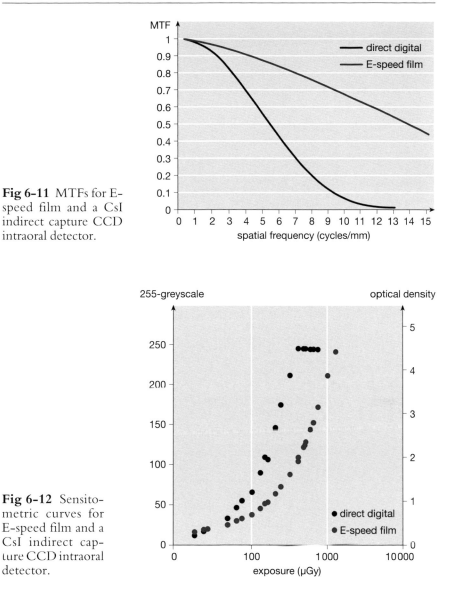

Fig 6-11 MTFs for E-speed film and a CsI indirect capture CCD intraoral detector.

Fig 6-12 Sensitometric curves for E-speed film and a CsI indirect capture CCD intraoral detector.

The exposure response of a detector is often expressed in terms of its characteristic curve (see Chapter 4), termed here the sensitometric curve. Fig 6-12 shows comparable sensitometric curves for a direct digital detector and Kodak E-speed film. The curves indicate that the digital detector requires less

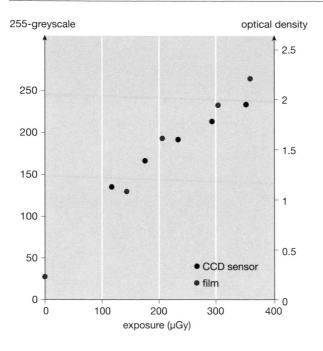

255-greyscale — optical density

CCD sensor
film

exposure (µGy)

Fig 6-13 Sensitometric curves for Kodak T-mat-L/RA dental film with Kodak lane regular screens and a scanning slot CCD sensor used in panoramic imaging.

radiation than film, up to 60% less in fact. The digital detector can be seen to saturate above 400 µGy and has a narrower latitude. It is important to note that this comparison is with E-speed film and not F-speed film. (At the time the data used in the figure were acquired, E-speed was the fastest film available.) The lower dose is achieved because the scintillator is more efficient at capturing the x-rays than the direct exposure film. However, if comparing with film–screen cassettes, as used in panoramic imaging, no dose saving is seen because both employ phosphor technology (Fig 6-13). Indeed, if a faster film–screen combination were used then a dose increase for a digital detector may be required. This is not unique in digital radiography and is accepted in order to achieve the benefits of digital, which include faster examinations and more efficient communication, image processing and digital storage.

The limited exposure latitude means that a direct digital sensor can produce underexposed or overexposed images in a similar way to film. The exposure kV response from a direct digital sensor is shown in Fig 6-14. "Auto ranging" on the images can reduce these effects, but it cannot compensate for lack of detector latitude.

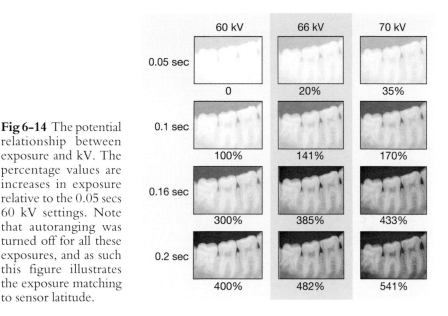

	60 kV	66 kV	70 kV
0.05 sec	0	20%	35%
0.1 sec	100%	141%	170%
0.16 sec	300%	385%	433%
0.2 sec	400%	482%	541%

Fig 6-14 The potential relationship between exposure and kV. The percentage values are increases in exposure relative to the 0.05 secs 60 kV settings. Note that autoranging was turned off for all these exposures, and as such this figure illustrates the exposure matching to sensor latitude.

Physical Characteristics

Whereas a phosphor image plate has many of the physical parameters of film, such as flexibility and size, direct digital sensors are bulkier. For example, a size 2 intraoral film is about 41 x 31 mm, yet the equivalent direct digital sensor is around 43 x 32 mm, with an active size of 36 x 26 mm (see Table 6-1, page 87), and it can be more than 6 mm in thickness. In addition, most sensors have a wire physically attached (Fig 6-15). It is important to note that because this is an electrical medical device attached to a patient it must be decoupled from the mains supply, so that if a system were damaged the patient would not be exposed to high voltages. One alternative to the wire is to use radio frequency communication with a wireless sensor (Fig 6-16). At the time of writing, one manufacturer has produced such a device, using a CMOS sensor, which is reported to have a battery life of around 500 exposures. For panoramic imaging, most detectors use long, thin sensors that fit behind the slit on the film holder. As the unit rotates around the patient the detector reads out multiple slices and stitches them into a single image.

Technical Considerations

There are several technical limitations to direct digital devices. Fig 6-17 is an image produced by exposure of the sensor without any intervening object.

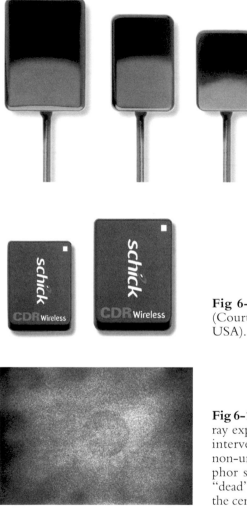

Fig 6-15 Direct digital intra-oral sensors. Three different sized sensors from the same manufacturer. (Courtesy of Schick Technologies, NY, USA).

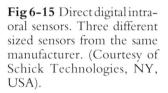

Fig 6-16 Wireless direct digital sensors. (Courtesy of Schick Technologies, NY, USA).

Fig 6-17 "Flat field" image obtained by x-ray exposure of the sensor with no object intervening. This shows low-frequency non-uniformity, probably from the phosphor structure. It is also possible to see "dead" pixels and a circular depression in the centre.

It shows a patch on the image, which is believed to arise from the phosphor structure, and a lot of inhomogeneity. Whereas the intensity and nature of this artefact should ensure it does not interfere with the clinical image, it is none the less an additional source of image noise. Another source of noise is "line structure" from the read out of the digital data. Fig 6-18 shows a strong line structure from a slot panoramic unit. Again, the intensity of the line structure is not high, but it could just be discerned on clinical images.

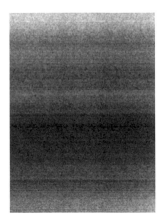

Fig 6-18 Line-structure artefact on a panoramic slot scanner.

This type of structured noise can often be subtracted out at the image acquisition stage. Another artefact that can occur is the "stitching artefact", which may appear where panels of detectors are stitched together. This is due to the software trying to interpolate inactive regions in the images, such as joins or dead pixels. This algorithm can in some instances show up in the clinical image (Fig 6-19). In this case, the manufacturer rewrote the interpolation algorithm and the artefact was removed.

Dead pixels can occur when the discrete pixel element in a sensor stops functioning. In Fig 6-17, some black points are visible which suggest dead pixels. Dead pixels are removed by interpolating the surrounding pixels to replace the missing elements in the final image. Structure noise is often removed by taking a flat field mask of the image, for example using Fig 6-17, and subtracting this from all subsequent images. Unfortunately, is not always evident when a sensor is failing, and interpolated signals, although improving the appearance of the image, are artificial points and may not relate to the actual anatomy. This is particularly an issue with large numbers or clusters of dead pixels.

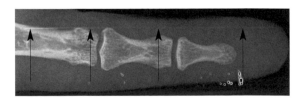

Fig 6-19 Example of a stitching artefact.

93

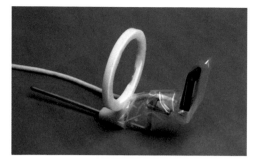

Fig 6-20 CCD-based sensor held in a suitable device to allow easier positioning and beam aiming. A simple plastic barrier is in place for cross-infection control.

Clinical Considerations

So far as intraoral systems are concerned, the main clinical issues with direct digital sensors relate to their physical size and the presence of the cable. Some patients find the sensors too large, which produces a gag reflex. Research has confirmed that there tends to be a higher retake rate with direct digital dental radiography. This is, of course, important in radiation dose terms because a retake would negate the dose advantage that these systems offer. Some improvement in ease of positioning during clinical use can be obtained by using sensor positioning aids. These are essentially the same as those used with film, but with suitable modifications to fix on to the sensor (Fig 6-20). The active area of sensors is also smaller than the physical size, and this can contribute to increased retake rates due to missed anatomy.

Patients may inadvertently bite into the sensor or wire. This may also occur with phosphor plates or film, of course, but the cost of a direct digital sensor is significantly higher if permanent damage occurs.

As with phosphor plates, barriers are required for cross-infection control and to avoid damage by saliva (Fig 6-20).

Further reading

Farman AG, Farman TT. A comparison of 18 different x-ray detectors currently used in dentistry. Oral Surg Oral Med Oral Pathol Oral Radiol Endod 2005;99(4):485–489.

Hell E, Knupfer W, Mattern D. The evolution of scintillating medical detectors. Nuclear Instruments and Methods in Physics Research Section A, 2000;454:40-48.

Litwiller D. CCD vs. CMOS: facts and fiction. Photonics Spectra 2001;35(1):154-158.

Van Der Stelt PF. Filmless imaging: The uses of digital radiography in dental practice. J Am Dent Assoc 2005;136:1379–1387.

Spartiotis K et al. A directly converting high-resolution intra-oral X-ray imaging sensor. Nuclear Instruments and Methods in Physics Research Section A, 2003;501:594-601.

Workman A, Brettle DS. Physical performance measures of radiographic imaging systems. Dentomaxillofac Radiol 1997;26(3):139–146.

Chapter 7
Indirect Digital Imaging

Aim

The aim of this chapter is to provide a comprehensive understanding of indirect digital x-ray imaging in dentistry.

Outcome

After reading this chapter the reader should be able to:
- describe the basic construction of a photostimulable phosphor plate
- explain how a typical indirect digital system works
- give the advantages and disadvantages of these systems.

What Does Indirect Digital Radiography Mean?

There is some confusion in the use of the term "indirect digital imaging". To some this means digitising a conventional radiograph using a flatbed scanner with a transparency adaptor. In this chapter, the term is used for images acquired using a photostimulable phosphor plate (PSP).

With these systems, once the PSP has been exposed the sensor has to be scanned by a laser before the image can be displayed. As there is this additional scanning process, these systems are referred to as indirect digital systems.

Principles of Indirect Digital Radiography
Construction of the PSP
The PSP is similar for all systems and comprises:
- a phosphor layer
- a reflective layer
- an electroconductive layer
- a polyester or polyethylene base layer
- a light-shielding layer
- protective layers.

A cross section of a PSP illustrating these layers and their functions is shown in Fig 7-1. A PSP will last for several thousand exposures, so long as it remains undamaged and free of scratches.

Interaction of the Phosphor Layer with X-radiation

When exposed to x-radiation, photoelectric interactions within the phosphor layer produce photoelectrons, which remove electrons from the europium activator. These electrons become trapped within fluorohalides at sites known as "F centres", leaving "holes" at the original europium sites. Some of the electrons drop back almost immediately, but importantly, the remaining electrons stay trapped within the F centres.

The number of trapped electrons at any particular point on the PSP is proportional to the original number of x-ray photons incident on that part of the sensor, thus producing a latent image.

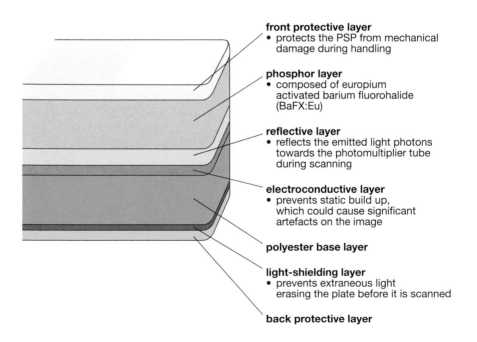

front protective layer
• protects the PSP from mechanical damage during handling

phosphor layer
• composed of europium activated barium fluorohalide (BaFX:Eu)

reflective layer
• reflects the emitted light photons towards the photomultiplier tube during scanning

electroconductive layer
• prevents static build up, which could cause significant artefacts on the image

polyester base layer

light-shielding layer
• prevents extraneous light erasing the plate before it is scanned

back protective layer

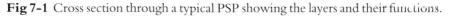

Fig 7-1 Cross section through a typical PSP showing the layers and their functions.

Scanning the PSP and Displaying the Image

The PSP with the stored latent image is scanned immediately using a thin red helium–neon laser beam. The laser energy causes the electrons to fall back into the europium holes, emitting light from the blue part of the visible spectrum. This process is known as "photostimulable luminence".

The blue light is detected by a photomultiplier tube (PMT). The PMT produces an amplified voltage proportional to the original light received. The voltage is converted into a digital signal by an analogue–digital converter (ADC). The ADC may have an output as high as 32 bits, which corresponds to over 4 billion grey level values. Because the human eye cannot perceive this many grey levels, the image is normally displayed with 256 shades of grey (8 bits).

Various scanning methods are employed, including the following:
* *Linear scanning.* The PSP is simply moved in front of a fixed laser source. The laser beam is deflected by mirrors onto the surface of the PSP. The Digora FMX and Optime (Soredex, Tuusala, Finland) use technology based on linear scanning.
* *Carousel/drum scanning.* The PSP is secured to a carousel, which rotates as the imaging head containing the laser moves down, parallel to the drum. The DenOptix (Gendex Dental Systems, Lake Zurich, USA) employs this method of scanning.
* *Spinner scanning.* The laser beam rotates while the PSP moves downwards. The laser is transmitted via a pentaprism onto the PSP. The blue light produced is reflected by parabolic mirrors onto the photomultiplier tubes. The VistaScan (Durr Dental, Beitigheim-Bissingen, Germany) employs spinner-type technology.

These scanning processes are shown in Fig 7-2 and examples of the equipment are shown in Fig 7-3.

Scanning times vary between systems. In addition, the scanning time may depend upon the scanning resolution selected, the size of the sensor being scanned and the number of sensors that require scanning. This time may be as short as 10 seconds for a single intraoral sensor, but for a "high-resolution" panoramic image it may be as long as 5 minutes.

Erasing the PSP

The Digora systems automatically erase the PSP during the scanning process, leaving it ready for immediate reuse. However, with the VistaScan and DenOptix systems a latent image remains after scanning. This is because

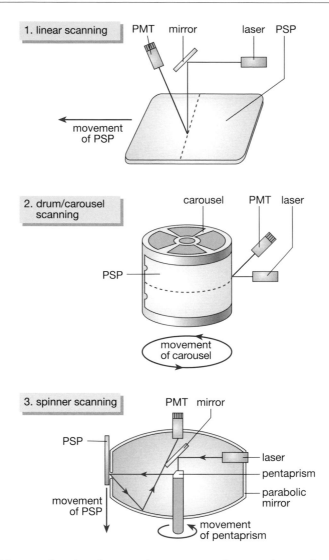

Fig 7-2 Diagram showing the scanning processes that may be employed by the indirect digital imaging systems; a) linear scanning; b) drum/carousel scanning; c) spinner scanning.

some of the electrons still remain within the F centres. Therefore, the sensor needs to be erased before being used again, otherwise a "double image" is produced. Erasure may be achieved by placing the PSP on a conventional

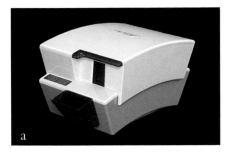
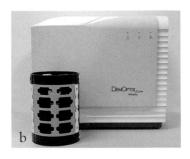
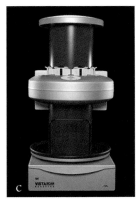

Fig 7-3 Examples of indirect digital imaging systems; a) Digora Optime, utilises linear scanning; b) Gendex DenOptix, utilises drum/carousel scanning; c) Dürr VistaScan, utilises spinner scanning.

light box. The time taken to erase the PSP will depend upon the intensity of the light produced (1000–5000 lux) but it should be cleared and ready for reuse in under 2 minutes. The PSP may also be erased using the manufacturer's dedicated erasure system.

A flow diagram showing these stages is given in Fig 7-4.

Physical Characteristics of the PSP

Conventional film used with intensifying screens shows a sigmoid shaped characteristic curve (Fig 7-5a). There is a background fog density, due mainly to plastic base. At each end of the curve there is a toe and shoulder. At these points large changes in exposure produce minimal changes in the optical density. It is only in the middle linear portion that small changes in exposure produce useful differences in density. Radiographic exposures are limited to this section of the curve – this is described as having a "narrow latitude".

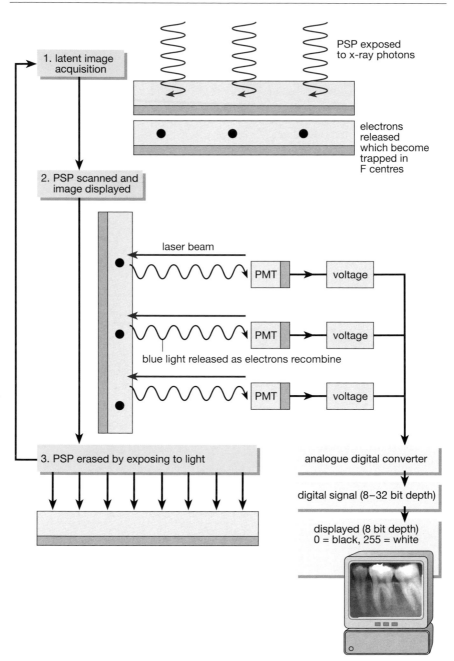

Fig 7-4 Diagram summarising how indirect digital images are acquired and displayed.

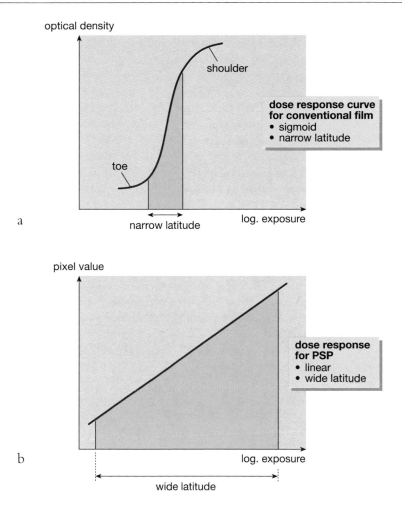

Fig 7-5 Graphs showing a) film characteristic curve for conventional film and b) the dose-response curve for a PSP.

With PSPs there is a wide latitude or dynamic range, because the response is linear over a wide range of exposures (Fig 7-5b). This allows both overexposed and underexposed images to be successfully displayed. However, at very low exposures, even though the image will still be displayed over an appropriate greyscale, there will be increased noise within the image, resulting in decreased image quality. It is for this reason that very low exposures cannot be used.

Radiation Dose

Diagnostically acceptable intraoral images may be obtained by reducing the dose by up to 50% in comparison with E-speed film. It may be that these dose reductions are not fully realised in practice because a low exposure setting may produce an image that is not as aesthetically pleasing to view. It is important at all times to keep the dose as low as possible without compromising the diagnostic yield.

The exposure factors used for extraoral views are similar to those used with conventional imaging with rare earth intensifying screens and medium film speed. Therefore, there is no, or minimal, dose reduction for these projections. It is important to realise this as these systems are often purchased in the belief that a significant dose reduction will be passed on to patients.

Taking an Intraoral Radiograph Using a "typical" System

1) The scanner should be located in the dental surgery according to the manufacturer's recommendations. In general, if the system does not have a daylight loading system then it should be positioned where the ambient lighting is below 1000 lux. This is necessary to ensure that the PSP is not erased before scanning.
2) The patient's details are entered into the software programme. The scanning resolution and the bit depth may also be adjusted before scanning.
3) The erased PSP is sealed in a single-use barrier envelope. This prevents possible cross-infection between patients and protects the PSP from incoming light and mechanical damage (Fig 7-6). The active surface of

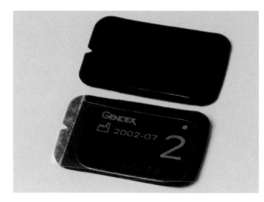

Fig 7-6 PSP in the barrier envelope. The envelope ensures that light does not erase the latent image before it is scanned. It also ensures the PSP is not contaminated by saliva.

the PSP is pale and the back surface is dark. It is important the PSP is placed in the barrier envelope correctly so that the active surface faces the x-ray source, otherwise a mirror image of the tooth will be produced.

4) The exposure is made. The PSP may be used with conventional film holders.

5) The barrier envelope is opened, and the PSP transferred to the scanner.

6) The PSP is scanned and the resultant image is displayed on the monitor.

Image Quality

One measure of image quality is the spatial resolution – the ability of the system to differentiate objects close together. This can be measured in line pairs per millimetre (lp/mm). The spatial resolution depends on many factors, including the scanning resolution – which is under direct control of the operator. It is also dependent upon the diameter of the scanning laser beam. The VistaScan uses a finer beam than other systems and this probably accounts for the higher resolution stated by the manufacturer. The resolution of direct action intraoral packet film can be as high as 20 lp/mm. The resolution of intraoral PSPs varies from system to system, but it is around 10 lp/mm. By and large, PSPs have a lower resolution than CCD and CMOS (solid-state) detectors (see Chapter 6).

Contrast resolution is a measure of how well objects with different attenuation coefficients can be distinguished from one another. This is probably as important clinically as the spatial resolution because it is important to be able to discriminate between tissues with only small differences in attenuation, such as early caries and the surrounding intact enamel. PSP systems generally have a lower contrast resolution compared with CCD and CMOS systems.

Advantages of Indirect Digital Radiography over Direct Digital Radiography

- *Size of active area of PSP.* As the phosphor coating covers the whole of the PSP, the active area is the same size as the sensor itself. The active area is generally greater than the equivalent size of CCD or CMOS detector. This means that fewer exposures may be necessary to image the required teeth, thus reducing the radiation dose (Fig 7-7).
- *Choice of PSPs.* There is a greater range of sensor sizes available, and therefore the optimum size of sensor can be chosen for each examination. Occlusal size PSPs are available. With the DenOptix and the VistaScan

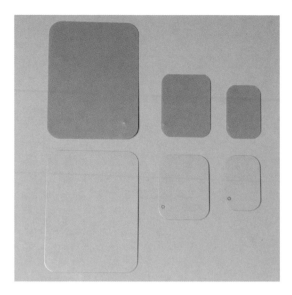

Fig 7-7 Typical range of sizes PSPs (lower row) showing they are of equivalent size to conventional film (upper row).

systems there is a choice of five intraoral PSPs (size 0–4 film equivalents). The Digora Optime has a choice of four sensor sizes (sizes 0–3 film equivalents). The occlusal size film (size 4) has to be scanned on a different unit – the Digora PCT system.

- *Conventional film holders may be used for intraoral radiography.* As the PSP has similar dimensions to conventional packet film then the operator's preferred choice of conventional film holder may be used, and so there is no period of learning to use new sensor holders (Fig 7-8). However, the PSP can become loose if the holder has been previously used for conventional film, as the film packet may be slightly thicker.

- *Intraoral PSP positioning and patient acceptance.* As there is no cable attached to the sensor, positioning of the PSP for intraoral radiography is relatively simple. As the PSP is easier for the patient to tolerate, the number of repeat radiographs is reduced.

- *Relatively low cost of PSPs.* Although the PSPs can be used several thousand times before having to be replaced, if an intraoral PSP becomes damaged then replacement is relatively inexpensive.

- *Wide latitude of exposure.* The PSP is much more tolerant than the CCD or CMOS sensors to changes in radiation exposure. As a result, both underexposure and overexposure will still produce images with adequate density. This means that if incorrect exposure factors were inadvertently used, it is less likely the examination would have to be repeated. How-

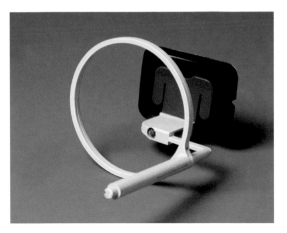

Fig 7-8 PSP in its barrier envelope placed in a conventional film holder.

ever, this feature does also have drawbacks as the operator may be unaware that the incorrect exposure factors have been selected and could continue to use these settings for further patients.

- *Existing extraoral x-ray equipment can be used.* For extraoral radiography the existing cassettes, with the intensifying screens removed, can be used to accommodate the PSPs. In addition, as the exposure times are generally similar to those used for conventional films, the x-ray machine does not need to be modified before use.
- *Less movement artefact on cephalometric views.* As the whole of the PSP is exposed at once there is less chance in producing movement artefacts.

Disadvantages of Indirect Digital Radiography compared with Direct Digital Radiography

- *Delay between exposure and image display.* There will always be a delay between exposure of the PSP and the image being displayed on the monitor. This delay is particularly relevant during endodontic therapy, when taking "working length" or "master cone" radiographs. Since treatment cannot proceed before these images are seen, there will be an inevitable, albeit slight, delay in treatment. However, it should be noted that these systems are still more rapid than conventional film processing.
- *Dose reduction.* For intraoral systems, greater dose reductions can be obtained using solid–state detectors compared with PSPs. There is no dose reduction at all using PSP extraoral imaging systems compared with conventional film/cassette based radiography.

107

- *Mechanical damage.* The PSP can be scratched or bent if not handled carefully (Fig 7-9). Forceps cannot be used to hold the PSP since these can permanently damage the sensor. Mechanical damage can also occur if the patient closes down onto the sensor, which can easily happen when taking occlusal views on children. Some manufacturers produce a guard that sandwiches and protects the sensor during occlusal radiography.
- *Image quality.* The spatial and contrast resolutions may not be as good as those of solid-state detectors. The images are, however, of sufficient quality for the diagnosis of dental disease.
- *Image "fogging".* If the PSP is exposed to a strong light source before scanning then the image could be erased or partially erased. A fully erased image appears white. A partially erased image can appear very grainy and with loss of detail (Fig 7-10b).
- *Double images.* On those systems where the PSP is not automatically erased during scanning it is possible to produce a double exposure if the operator inadvertently forgets to erase the PSP before reusing it. This mistake cannot happen with those systems based on CCD or CMOS technology (Fig 7-10e).
- *PSP flexibility.* Having a thin PSP does mean increased patient tolerance, but this flexibility could lead to image distortion if the sensor is bent during the exposure (Fig 7-10f).

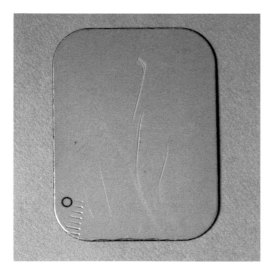

Fig 7-9 Damaged PSP. These marks would produce white artefacts on the image.

Fig 7-10 PSP images demonstrating some of the drawbacks of the system; a) original image; b) image if the PSP is partially erased due to light exposure before scanning; c) image if a scratched sensor is used, showing the characteristic white marks; d) image if the PSP is inadvertently placed back to front, producing a mirror image; e) image if the PSP is not erased before being reused, producing a double image; f) image if the sensor is bent in the mouth, producing distortion of the image. Note the distortion in the trabeculae above the roots of the teeth.

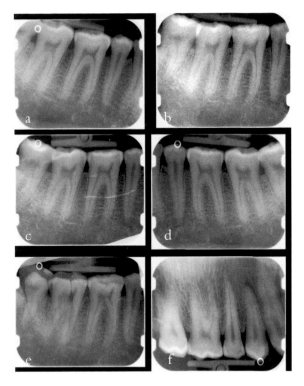

Key Points

- Indirect digital systems always involve a scanning stage before the image can be seen.
- PSPs may be used several thousand times, but they must be carefully looked after since if scratched they need to be replaced.
- There is a wide latitude of exposure, so underexposed or overexposed images are usually displayed with the correct density.
- Image quality is acceptable for clinical use.
- For intraoral radiography there may be a dose reduction in comparison with E-speed film, but there is no significant dose reduction on extraoral views.

Further Reading

Hildebolt CF, Couture RA, Whiting BR. Dental photostimulable phosphor radiography. Dent Clin North Am 2000;44(2):273–297.

Oakley J. Digital Imaging: a primer for radiographers, radiologists and health care professionals. London: Greenwich Medical Media, 2003, Ch. 3, pp 17–50.

Smith B, Burns B, Carlton R. Digital radiography. In: Carlton RR, Adler AM (eds). Principles of Radiographic Imaging; an art and a science. 3rd edn. Albany, NY: Delmar, 2001, pp 632-649.

Chapter 8

Image Storage and Handling

Aim

The aim of this chapter is to provide an understanding of the methods of image storage and handling, and in particular to provide knowledge of the rather complex terminology associated with the subject.

Outcome

After reading this chapter, the reader should understand:
- the terminology used by manufacturers and technical support services, to ensure they are getting the correct equipment, specification and support
- the basic elements involved in image handling, including communications standards, computer networking, image display and image storage.

Introduction

In digital imaging systems, acquisition and display are not intrinsically linked, as with a film system, but are separated. This enables almost unlimited and highly efficient storage, communication and display of the digital data. However, the success or failure of a digital imaging system rests on the correct set-up of each of the many technical elements comprising it. This chapter focuses on this challenging subject. It does not cover application software, as there are many products available, each with their own nuances. Needless to say, a user evaluation of any software before purchase is essential.

There are two main methodologies for handling digital dental images. The first is to use dedicated "standalone" systems, which are often proprietary systems based around a personal computer. They are used for single-modality applications, such as a single intraoral camera or a single CCD x-ray detector. This type of system is common in dental applications (Fig 8-1). In addition to the basic computer functions of display and short-term storage, they often have a method for long-term storage, such as a DVD or CD writer, and the ability to print good quality images. The limiting factor with these systems is that they have no, or very limited, connectivity and communication with other systems.

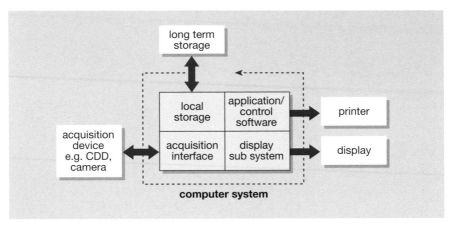

Fig 8-1 Standalone single-modality system, where the core functions of image handling are combined in one computer.

The second methodology is the "distributed" system (Fig 8-2), which has dedicated systems for each function. This allows multi-modality and multiple users to share the same system. This type of system is generically referred to as a picture archival and communication system (PACS) or mini PACS, and is usually installed in larger institutions.

Regardless of the terminology or size, all these systems are effectively PACSs as they will archive and communicate pictures. Most systems will also use generic building blocks that are as applicable to a small system as they are to a larger one.

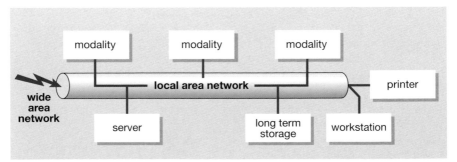

Fig 8-2 Distributed image handling, with dedicated systems for each function.

Medical Radiography Standards

The whole field of digital imaging in medicine is developing at an increasing rate, not only with respect to the modality and associated technologies but also with respect to the development of standards. Two standards are currently key to the integration of medical imaging systems; the Digital Imaging and Communications in Medicine (DICOM) and the Health Level Seven (HL7) standards.

DICOM

What is DICOM? DICOM is a ratified standard from the American College of Radiologists (ACR) and the National Electronics Manufacturers Association (NEMA) that aims to standardise connectivity in medical imaging. The need for this arose with the advent of digital imaging where each manufacturer would have their own method of connectivity and image storage. The current level of DICOM is version 3 although this is a little misleading as the previous version was called the ACR/NEMA standard 2.0. Additionally, although version 3 was released in 1993, there are frequent additions to the DICOM standard by the use of supplements. Most, if not all, manufacturers of medical imaging equipment now adhere to DICOM version 3. This does not, however, ensure compatibility of equipment, and terms such as "DICOM compatible" and "DICOM enabled" may be erroneous. DICOM at the technical level is quite complex; the perception that DICOM specification is difficult is further enhanced by DICOM conformance statements, which are impenetrable technical documents often issued at the tender stage by manufacturers and not really appropriate for clinical end users. This section aims to demystify DICOM and provide a practical level of knowledge to assist in purchasing decisions and in the day-to-day use of DICOM modalities. For those who wish to learn more about DICOM there is an official DICOM website (http://medical.nema.org), and the website of David Clunie is an excellent DICOM resource: (http://www.dclunie.com).

DICOM service classes
The service classes can be thought of as the DICOM communications protocols. They specify the levels of connectivity between modalities. The seven most useful classes for medical imaging are:
• Verification
• Modality Work List
• Performed Procedure Step
• Store

113

- Storage Commit
- Print
- Query/Retrieve.

Not all these classes may be available on all modalities, and may be conditional on whether the service class is being used or provided by the modality. With each DICOM communication, a communication exchange is set up; where one system is the user and the other the provider. Therefore, in specifying DICOM service classes you have to decide your role: whether you just want to use that service (service class user – SCU), provide it (service class provider – SCP), or both.

An example of a DICOM communication would be where a modality wants to store an image on another modality: the sender will have to have DICOM Store at the SCU level and the receiver will have to have DICOM Store at the SCP level.

The sender could also receive images to store, but this would be a separate communication and would require DICOM Store SCP as well. A list of the service classes and the user/provider context is shown in Table 8-1.

DICOM object
The DICOM object is the part of DICOM that contains the image data. This will contain not just the images but also all other modality-specific information to ensure the receiving system knows how the image is formatted and presented. There are many DICOM objects, and new ones are being added all the time. The current list includes, for example:
CR = computed radiography
CT = computed tomography
MR = magnetic resonance
NM = nuclear medicine
US = ultrasound
RG = radiographic imaging (conventional film/screen)
DX = digital radiography
MG = mammography
IO = intraoral radiography
PX = panoramic x-ray.

From this list it can be seen that dental-specific modalities are included. In many respects, the end-user does not need to be concerned with this level of DICOM other than to ensure that the relevant service class, roles and

Table 8-1 **DICOM service classes.** SCU = service class user; SCP = service class provider

		Service class role		
		SCU	SCP	SCU and SCP
DICOM service classes	*Verification*	Can check to see if a DICOM communication is possible on another system	Can accept a DICOM communication check request to provide the required service	Can check and confirm that DICOM communications are possible
	Modality work list	Radiological information system (RIS) – sends a work list to the modality	Modality – can receive work lists from the RIS	N/A
	Performed procedure step	Modality can send confirmation to the RIS that an examination is complete	RIS – can receive confirmation that an examination is complete	N/A
	Store	Can send images to storage	Can receive images to store	Can send and receive images to storage
	Storage commit	Can transfer ownership of images to the store modality	Can take ownership of images from the send modality	Can assign or receive ownership of images with another modality
	Print	Can send images to print	Can receive images to print	Can send and receive images to print
	Query/ retrieve	Can query a remote database and retrieve images from it	Allows its database to be queried and images retrieved	Can query and retrieve from another database and allows others to query retrieve its own database

object are supported. This can be specified by using the DICOM service object pair (SOP).

DICOM service object pair
We have defined the service class, the service class role and the object; we can now use these to specify the exact DICOM functionality of the modality using the DICOM SOP. The SOP should be stated in a modality specification and used to establish levels of DICOM communication. An example would be a simple digital x-ray unit that can store to PACSs only.

The SOP for the modality would be:

Service class	Role	SOP
Store	SCU	DX

whereas the SOP for the PACS would be:

Service class	Role	SOP
Store	SCP	DX, US, MR, CT, etc.

The end-user looking at these SOPs can see that the two systems are compatible for the purpose of DICOM Store.

Modality configuration
The preceding sections dealt with the theory and specification of DICOM connectivity. An equally important element is the physical set-up of the modalities. Each modality has to be uniquely identified on the network. This is achieved in three ways: the IP address, the Application Entity Title and the port number:

- *IP address.* The IP (Internet Protocol) address is a unique four-part numerical identifier. The range of IPs is unique for a particular network, and an individual unique IP is issued by the network administrator for each modality. A typical IP could be 192.168.120.5; IP addresses are covered in more detail in the section on networking.
- *Application entity title (AET).* The AET is effectively the name of the modality on the network. A usual syntax would be AET_MXRRM1; which stands for main x-ray (MXR) room 1 (RM1). AETs can be extremely useful in administration tasks as they allow modalities to be identified without the need to refer to lookup tables. However, ambiguous AETs, such as AET_A012DFRZ1, can cause delays in fault finding, particularly on large systems. Additionally, errors can be introduced in having to retype

complex AETS, as these may need to be entered on all devices that the modality needs to connect to. Some DICOM modalities allow verified DICOM identities to be turned off. This allows them to accept any DICOM connection, which can be advantageous in some cases, but in general verified DICOM identities are preferable.

- *Port number.* Computers connected to a network have a number of virtual ports that they can access (see the section on networking). These can be thought of as numbered subconnections on the computer. If a port is closed, no connection is available. Additionally, if the software is listening to the wrong port, it will not recognise when a DICOM communication is taking place. Therefore, the correct port, which has been specified in the local DICOM settings, must also be specified on other modalities. It does not matter which port number is used as long as it is specified at both ends of the communication. Ports 104 and 4006 are often used for DICOM purposes; one model could use port 104 for workstations and port 4006 for modalities, or 4006 for all DICOM devices.

DICOM greyscale standard display function (Part 14)
There are additional DICOM components that are of a more specialised nature and not of interest to the general reader. However, one additional component is essential to the correct display of images: the DICOM greyscale standard display function (GSDF).

There is a huge choice of commercial displays, each with its own characteristics. This is not helpful for viewing medical images, as an image on one monitor may appear completely different on another monitor. The DICOM GSDF was defined in an attempt to standardise image display. The GSDF describes the non-linear human perceptual response to different levels of luminance. It is based on a model of the human visual system and defines a standard curve against which different types of display devices can be calibrated. In this way, the calibrated image display uses the available contrast of the display device in a "perceptually" linear way (i.e. the difference between black and 5% grey is perceived equal to the difference between white and 95% grey). This calibration can yield a consistent image display, which means that the appearance of the image to the human observer is as similar as possible given the differing properties of display devices.

To set up the DICOM display function correction requires the measurement of the characteristic curve of a display system. This is done using a number of uniform images with areas of constant grey level from black to white and a photometer. A lookup table (LUT) is generated by mapping

117

each point on the GSDF curve to the closest point on the measured curve. This LUT is then used to map the measured characteristic curve to the GSDF. This task can often be conducted automatically on high-end monitors, and lower specification monitors often have built-in DICOM curves applied.

Health Level Seven (HL7)

Although DICOM is a key component in a PACS, the system still requires integration with the patient management system to ensure that images are unambiguously linked to the correct patient. This is achieved using information system standards such as HL7.

HL7 is a standard that is accredited by the American National Standards Institute (ANSI) to provide a standardised method of interfacing hospital information systems. This is very much a standard for system integrators and developers, and for the large part the clinical user will be unaware of HL7 except when procuring information systems or PACSs. However, it is a pivotal component in PACSs as it ensures consistency of data, theoretically all the way from the hospital information system (HIS) or practice management software, through to the radiological information system (RIS) – in larger institutions – and through to the modality. This then ensures that any image data acquired at the modality is intrinsically linked to high probity demographics from the initial booking stage.

This has two major benefits; first, workflow at the modality is faster as the patient will automatically be listed through DICOM work lists, making entry of data at the modality unnecessary; and second, the instances of unvalidated images will be reduced or eliminated. Unvalidated images can occur if patient demographics are incorrectly entered at any stage; for example, if a patient's correct name is "Stephens" but at the modality it is spelt "Stevens" there will be a mismatch of the data. This can result in either the data being rejected by a PACS, as it will not match the HIS data, or duplicate entries being generated for the same patient. As a result, either the images will not be available to view, until they are manually fixed to the HIS database, or only some or no images will be retrieved when searching for the patient on the image database at a later date.

Networking

A major component in any digital image system, particularly with multi modalities and workstations, is the network.

In a multi-surgery dental practice there may be several computers and associated x-ray systems, linked by a network. A computer network is not just the physical connection between computers, it also includes the communication protocols running on it. The following is a simple introduction to the most common components and terminology encountered in setting up a digital imaging network. The basic principles will be the same, from a simple peer-to-peer, computer-to-computer connection through to a hospital-wide corporate system. There are many sources of information on networking, including the Internet, and the UK MHRA Evaluation Centre PACSNet has produced a useful background document for healthcare users in the UK (see Further Reading).

There are two general categories of network, the local area network (LAN) and the wide area network (WAN):
* a LAN is usually small scale, for a single building or group of buildings, e.g. a large dental practice or hospital site (Fig 8-3)

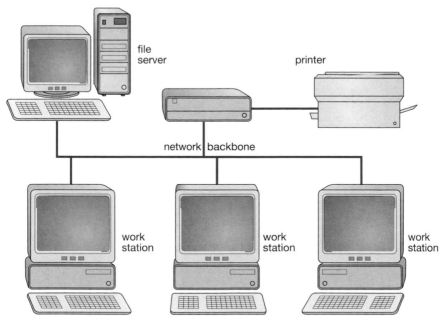

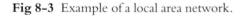

local area network (LAN)

Fig 8-3 Example of a local area network.

- a WAN (Fig 8-4) covers a wide area, such as the Internet. An example could be a network covering all the sites owned by a corporate provider of dental services, each of which would have its own LAN. The Internet is effectively a world-wide WAN as it is constructed of a network of networks.

A third term that is frequently used is storage area network (SAN). This is not a network model in its own right, rather it refers to the ability to have storage anywhere on a network, not just at the servers. A SAN can be thought of as storage elements on a network: the servers communicate with the storage elements, termed network attached storage (NAS), as if they were locally attached drives. This could be, for example, a large RAID (see section on storage, below) for central storage.

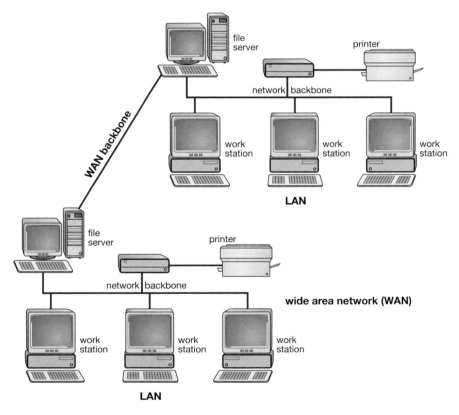

Fig 8-4 Example of a wide area network.

When a network has more than one connection there is a need for hardware to handle the network traffic. There are several different components that can be used; these are hubs, switches, routers and bridges.

Hubs, Switches, Routers and Bridges

The key components in any network are the hubs, switches, routers and bridges. Often, one device can have the functionality of several of these single devices.

- *Hub.* A hub is a common connection for devices in a network and allows segments of a LAN to be connected. This is achieved through ports, which are the connections to the hub for each segment. When a packet (a small block of data) arrives at one port, it is copied to the other ports so that all segments of the LAN can see all the network packets.
- *Switch.* A switch can be thought of as an intelligent hub. It is also a connector between two or more computers' data, which allows them to communicate with each other to form a LAN. The switch reads the IP address for the data destination and sends the data to the relevant port only.
- *Router.* A router is a connector between two or more networks to allow them to communicate with each other to form a WAN. A router works at the IP level and makes decisions about which of several paths network (or Internet) traffic will follow.
- *Bridge.* A bridge is a device for network data control that works at a hardware level, using a computer's MAC address (see Ethernet, below) to communicate (Fig 8-5). An example of this would be where a computer had two network cards installed, working on two different LANs; the PC could then be set to be a bridge across the two networks, using the network card MAC addresses. This could also be achieved using a physical device, but the advantage of a bridge is that it can be moved anywhere on the bridged network and still function without reconfiguration.

Ethernet

Ethernet is one of the most popular network protocols for LANs. It is based at the physical level on wired connections between computers. There are two types of wiring, coaxial and twisted pair, although coaxial is not often used as it is slower (10 Mbit/s) than the thinner twisted pair, which in its current format (Cat 5e+) can achieve 1 Gbit/s. This is more than adequate for most image networks, and 100 Mbit/s to the desktop is often sufficient. Because of its popularity it is cheap to implement and many PCs already come with Gbit network connectivity enabled.

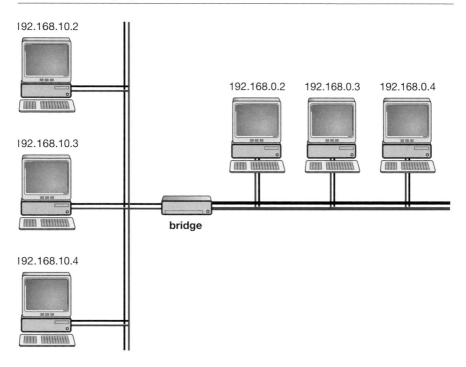

Fig 8-5 Example of a bridge between two different networks.

Above the physical level, Ethernet communicates between computers by sending packets, which are small blocks of data. Each Ethernet connection is given a 48-bit MAC address (machine address), which is used to uniquely identify the connection for both sending and receiving data.

WiFi
WiFi refers to wireless networking. This allows the physical limitations of network wiring to be overcome. However, WiFi has limitations over a dedicated wired network. The first limitation is the range. This is very dependent on where the devices are installed, but certainly walls will reduce the range. The second limitation is that the speed of a wireless network is slower than a wired one. The network speed, which is dependent on the WiFi standard used and the signal strength, may be a significant issue for the transfer of large numbers of large images. The WiFi standard 802.11b is the slowest at 11 Mbit/s, the 802.11g maximum is 54 Mbit/s, and the proposed 802.11n will be the fastest with a theoretical 540 Mbit/s. The third limitation

is that there are still concerns about the security of wireless connections; they are theoretically easier to "snoop" on or to access than wired networks. Encryption and connection validation methods can make WiFi networking more secure but from a pure quality of service perspective wired networks are preferable to wireless ones.

TCP/IP

There are various models for networking; one of the most commonly used is the TCP/IP. It is based on four layers:

- *Layer 1:* The physical link. Commonly based on Ethernet.
- *Layer 2:* The network protocol. This is the component that sends the data from end to end in packets; often it is the Internet Protocol (IP). The location of each end of the data transfer is specified in an IP address. This is constructed of four bytes, e.g. 192.168.0.5. IP addresses are often allocated in ranges, e.g. 192.168.0.1–192.168.0.128. In addition to the IP address is the subnet mask. This is used in conjunction with the IP address to identify the user number. In many networks the IP address is dynamically allocated using the dynamic host configuration protocol (DHCP), however in imaging networks these addresses are often static as a fixed relationship is required.
- *Layer 3:* Transport: the transmission control protocol (TCP) and the user datagram protocol (UDP). The IP protocol can get corrupted as packets get corrupted. In order to control this, the UDP adds checksums and also port access to ensure correct application association. TCP protocol streams the packets to ensure the data arrives at the application in the correct order.
- *Layer 4:* Application. The software using the network communication.

These protocols can operate independently on the operating systems of the connection computers.

Display

In chapters 6 and 7 we concentrated on the technology and practicalities of acquiring the information contained in the x-ray beam. For the dentist, the "bottom line" is the viewing of images in a clinical context, and here we must consider the relative value of soft and hard copies.

Soft Copy

Soft copy display is the ability to view images without permanently recording them onto a transport medium, such as film or paper. This is usually achieved by viewing images on a monitor. Currently, there are two main technology groups suitable for soft copy monitors; the cathode ray tube (CRT) and flat panel displays. Whereas the CRT is a specific technology, flat panel display encompasses a number of very different technologies. Medical imaging is one of the most demanding applications for display technologies. Each different technology has its own pros and cons and should be carefully considered before use in medical imaging applications.

Although the display monitor is a crucial element in any soft copy display system, it is often the last element considered, if it is considered at all. This situation is worsening with the increase in remote viewing of images, often on PC-based systems via web servers, where there is limited or no control over the display used. Considering the costs involved in acquiring images in the first place it should be of concern that these images may end up being viewed on monitors that have not been selected for suitability, have not been optimised and undergo no quality assurance.

CRT
The CRT was developed by Ferdinand Braun, a German scientist, in 1897, but it was not used in the first television sets until the late 1940s. Although the CRTs found in modern monitors have undergone modifications to improve picture quality, they still follow the same basic principles as the 1897 design. The main advantage of a CRT is that it is a mature technology that can deliver high-luminance, high-fidelity images that have a natural appearance. Furthermore, as it is an emissive device, a CRT screen can be viewed at any angle and a consistent image is visible. The main disadvantages are that it has a high power consumption (and as such runs hot), is prone to geometric distortions across the screen and emits strong magnetic and electromagnetic fields. They are also physically heavy and large. CRTs have now been effectively replaced in the medical display market by the improving flat panel displays.

Flat panel display
The flat panel display category includes a number of very different technologies, such as liquid crystal displays (LCD), plasma displays, organic light-emitting diodes (OLED) and various other devices. Within these technologies, one can distinguish between flat panel displays that emit light (emissive devices) and those with a backlight that passes light through them (transmissive).

Currently, the most useful displays for medical imaging are those based on LCD technology. A TFT-LCD display comprises three main components: the backlight, the liquid crystal sandwich and the thin-film transistors. The transistors allow a pixel matrix to be defined such that each pixel can be addressed and controlled individually, allowing the image to be constructed (Fig 8-6). The main limitations of a transmissive device are:

- the viewing angle is restricted; the image contrast is affected when viewed at an acute angle to the image plane
- individual transistors on the TFT can fail, resulting in fixed on or off pixels
- the backlight can fade or be non-uniform.

Another important factor with LCD displays is that the pixels are in a fixed location, which defines the physical matrix size of the display – termed the "native resolution". If a resolution lower than the native resolution is used, the electronics will scale the "smaller" image up to the maximum size of the display panel. If the circuitry cannot handle this task efficiently, the result will be distorted and poor quality. Such digital displays should always be used at their native resolution.

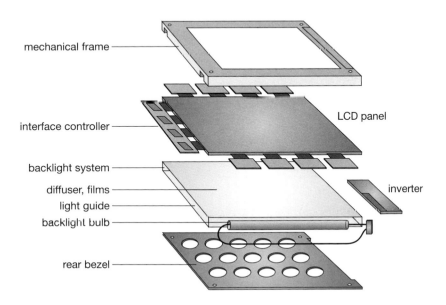

Fig 8-6 Composition of a TFT–LCD display.

CRT vs TFT-LCD

It used to be the case that one of the first issues with respect to a potential purchase is whether the display should be a CRT or LCD device. There have, however, been several recent publications comparing the technical and diagnostic performance of CRT and LCD displays that have suggested that current TFT-LCD displays may be suitable for soft copy reporting, and that they may even be better than CRTs due to lower veiling glare and isotropic modulation transfer function. It is important though to understand the limitations of the technology, such as the restricted viewing angle, in order to achieve optimal display. If these concerns are considered, there does not appear to be any major technological reason for not using a TFT-LCD display for all display requirements.

Other factors may affect the choice of display, such as size, weight, heat output and magnetic field considerations. It is also important to note that a comparable specification CRT will produce a more "film-like" image than its TFT-LCD counterpart due to its analogue nature and that LCD displays must be driven at their native resolution.

Location of monitors

The positioning of monitors has to be carefully considered in order to minimise reflections and ambient light sources, which are a significant factor in image degradation. Positioning displays facing windows or other strong light sources, such as light boxes or lamps, should be avoided. In areas with high ambient light or reflections, high-luminance monitors are advantageous, as is the use of monitor hoods. Use of software contrast and brightness controls may compensate for loss of contrast, although this may not be practicable in some environments, such as in operating theatres. Hardware brightness and contrast controls must not be used as these may compromise any DICOM calibration.

Monitor selection

Selecting the correct monitor display is not as straightforward as it might seem; there are many different manufacturers supplying a wide range of displays, and selecting suitability for purpose is a difficult task. One proposed approach is to use a banding scheme, by which an application can be matched to a band of equipment, selected by stratifying a manufacturer's product line. Such a scheme is shown in Table 8-2.

Once a band has been selected, the minimum technical specification needs to be set. There are three main components in this respect: monitor size,

Table 8-2 **Banding scheme for soft copy displays used in hospital applications** (Table from Brettle, 2007).

Band	Description	Example
A+	Highest end reporting for demanding applications	Mammography
A	High-quality reporting monitor	Radiology conventional reporting
B	Reporting monitor for lower contrast or resolution modalities or highly supportive review applications e.g. immediate feedback to clinical activity	MR, PET, CT, US, cardiology
C	Review monitor not to be used for diagnosis; images to be viewed only in conjunction with the report	Ward, clinic
D	Do not use to view clinical images	IT only applications

matrix size and luminance range. To a large degree the selection can be dictated by the viewing constraints, such as distance from monitor, ambient light conditions and diagnostic task.

Ambient lighting
The American Association of Physicists in Medicine (AAPM) Task Group 18 report (2005) gives details on maximum levels for ambient light, depending on the minimum luminance of the monitor and the reflectivity of the surface. These are summarised in Table 8-3.

Monitor viewing distance
It stands to reason that the further away the monitor is, the larger it has to be if the effective size is to be the same. It is not just the physical size of the monitor that matters, but also the number of pixels available to display the image. Table 8-4 shows the distances from a monitor required to resolve a 1 mm separation. This is shown for three typical monitor configurations and will allow you to select a monitor that fits with your surgery layout.

Table 8-3 **Maximum room lighting (lux) based on AAPM Task Group 18 Report.** (It should be noted that the IPEM Report 91 specifies a room illumination not greater than 15 lux for reporting areas).

Monitor luminance (cd/m²)		Diffuse reflectivity coefficient		
L_{max}	L_{min}	Low (0.01)	Mid (0.02)	High (0.03)
250	1	25	12.5	6.25
500	2	50	25	12.5
1000	4	100	50	25
2000	10	250	125	62.5
5000	20	500	250	125

Table 8-4 **Maximum viewing distances for three typical monitor configurations.** (Maximum viewing distance is the distance at which it is possible to resolve 1 mm for the same image displayed at full resolution).

Resolution (pixels)	Mega pixels	Diagonal size (inches)	Pixel size (mm)	Maximum viewing distance (cm)
1200 x 1024	1.2	17	0.264	343
1600 x 1200	2	19	0.22	381
2048 x 1536	3	21	0.21	463

Soft copy quality assurance

After installing a digital x-ray system in the practice, many of us probably do no more aftercare than the occasional wipe of the monitor screen with a duster or damp cloth. In the UK, the Institute of Physics and Engineering in Medicine (IPEM) Report 91 specifies a series of quality assurance tests for soft copy display. These tests are split into two groups: type A and type B. Type A tests are intended to be done by local users daily or every three months; these include image display condition, the ratio of black to white levels in the image, and resolution and distance calibration where appropriate. The more detailed type B tests are conducted every 6-12 months and include checking the display greyscale, GSDF uniformity, variation between monitors and the room illumination.

To conduct these tests requires a photometer and a test image. The test image can be a simple SMPTE (Fig 8-7) or DICOM TG18-QC image and can be downloaded from the Internet, generated by dedicated software or pre-installed on the system. If pre-installed, it is important to ensure the image is a high-quality version.

Photometers can be split into two main types: telescopic hand-held types and near-range, contact probes (Fig 8-8). The latter are the simplest to use, and they currently cost around £1000.

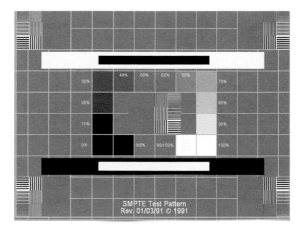

Fig 8-7 SMPTE test image used for routine quality assurance, as specified by the IPEM Report 91.

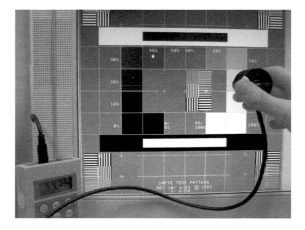

Fig 8-8 A contact probe photometer. (Photograph courtesy of Elizabeth Arnott and Craig Munnings).

129

Cleaning and infection control
All displays need to be regularly cleaned to remove dust and fingerprints. In the dental surgery, however, it is also necessary to consider infection control. It is possible that the various cleaning products and surface disinfectants used in a clinical environment might damage the polymer or antireflective surface supplied on many displays. Where there is no chance of contamination of the display by body fluids, all that is necessary is that the manufacturer's recommendations for cleaning are placed on the display casing.

For areas of low infection risk it may be acceptable to specify "wipe clean" for surfaces such as glass fronts for displays, again with appropriate cleaning protocols specified. Where there is a significant infection risk, conformance is required to the IP65 level, which provides protection to the level that dust can not enter at all and water jets directed at the enclosure from any direction must not have any harmful effect.

Hard Copy
Hard copy is the process of permanently recording an image to a transport medium, such as film. While there will be no need to make routine hard copies of digital images, there will be times when hard copies are required, such as when referring patients to colleagues. There are currently four main technologies for hard copy recording of digital dental images; inkjet, thermal, laser paper and laser film.

Inkjet
Inkjet technology can provide high-quality images onto either a film base or a paper base. Although consumer models will only allow for a low throughput, modified printers with large external ink tanks can provide for a reasonable workload. It is important to note that for best prints grey inks should be used rather than coloured inks. Inkjet images are not water resistant, and unless archive quality media and inks are used the images will fade. Pigment inks provide for better archiving quality than dye inks. The cost per print can also be high.

Thermal
Thermal printing has been used for medical applications for many years in applications such as ultrasound imaging. However, the quality is relatively poor and the images will fade with time. In addition, if the print gets hot it will fade more quickly. On balance it is not the best technology, other than perhaps for patient copies.

Laser paper
Commercial laser paper printers have continued to improve in terms of quality and cost. Many new models have greyscale printing capabilities and may be a viable solution for many applications. However, unless an acetate base is used the images are reflection only, and using an acetate base for transmission images produces lower quality prints.

Laser film
Currently, dedicated medical-grade laser imagers are the only recommended *diagnostic* grade hardcopy device for digital images. The images are very high quality, have good archive properties and are transmission images. They are the closest solution to producing traditional films from digital data. In addition, most laser imagers should have DICOM Print and so can be networked, providing a total solution for digital dental imaging. The main downside is the cost of these units, both in terms of the purchase cost of the imager and the film costs. Additionally, there is currently no imager that will print intraoral "films" onto standard size prints. Therefore, the cost per print for intraoral images will be high if an 18 x 24 cm film is used for a 3 x 4 cm intraoral image.

Storage

Integrity and robustness of data storage are essential for a digital radiographic image system. The two main levels of storage are local and tertiary. The local storage is often the modality storage; the local space where the modality puts its images before transferring them to the main archive. This is fast storage to maximise workflow, usually a hard disc drive (HDD). In a small single-modality system, such as a small dental practice, this may also be the long-term storage. The tertiary archive can be slower than the local storage, but it needs to be larger, especially if long-term multi-modality storage is required. In reality there may be three levels of storage, the primary modality archive, the central (PACS) on-line secondary archive (e.g. RAID) and the tertiary storage for the central archive (e.g. tape library).

- The primary storage is the fastest to access and is always on-line but is usually limited in size.
- The secondary storage is much larger than the primary and may also be on-line, but it will be slower to access than the primary archive.
- The tertiary storage may be on-line, but it is usually near-line or off-line. This means that images have to be loaded before they can be retrieved; near-line storage is usually a "jukebox", where a tape is retrieved by a

robotic arm, and off-line would be where the tape needs to be loaded by a human after retrieving it from a deep store.

It is important to ensure that not only is the image data stored in a backup, but also the image location database is updated. This database is equally as important as the image data.

When designing storage systems, one of the primary design concerns is to remove "single points of failure" (SPF). One hard disc in a single-modality system is a SPF. This risk can be reduced by using a RAID (see below) and a backup, e.g. CD, DVD or tape. This chapter can not cover all the archive technologies available as these change rapidly as new technologies mature. Instead, an introduction to RAID options and backup strategies will be given; it will be assumed that a suitable technology for the purpose will be used.

RAID
RAID is an acronym for "redundant array of independent/inexpensive disks". A RAID is a means of using multiple discs to either increase the speed of data access or increase the robustness of an archive, or both. To the end-user there will appear to be only one disk drive. RAID used to be used in high-end data-critical applications, however this function is now supplied on low-cost computers. It does require at least two hard discs depending on the level of RAID required. There are several levels of RAID, but a detailed analysis is beyond the scope of this text; for more detail, online reference sources offer a good overview.

The two most commonly implemented methods are outlined below.
RAID 1: Mirroring (Fig 8-9)
• Requires a minimum of two discs.
• The data is written simultaneously to each disc.
• Has the advantage that if a single disc fails the data can be rebuilt from the other.
• Offers redundancy, but not any speed improvement. It can take time to rebuild the new disc, during which time the system will be unavailable.

RAID 10: Stripping and mirroring (Fig 8-10)
• Effectively RAID 1 (mirroring of data) with RAID 0 (stripping of data).
• Requires a minimum of four discs.
• Offers high redundancy with improvement in read times as parity does not need to be calculated.
• The system can survive all but one discs failing in each RAID 1.

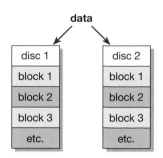

Fig 8-9 Example of how data is written with RAID 1.

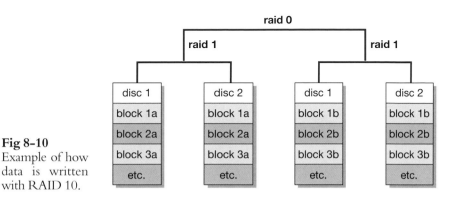

Fig 8-10
Example of how data is written with RAID 10.

RAID 1 (mirroring) is recommended as a minimum for single-modality systems, and for larger systems, where service continuity is required, RAID 10 (stripping and mirroring) is recommended. The size of a RAID can vary enormously, from two discs to hundreds, and archives with many terrabytes of storage are now cost-effective solutions for the end-user.

Backup Strategies

There are several standard strategies for data backup. These include:
- *Full-system backups,* where all the data on the server is written to removable media, making a full complete record of the system.
- *Incremental backups,* which only backs up files that have changed since the last full backup, this is used in conjunction with a full backup.
- *Mirror backup,* where a complete replica of the sever is kept on permanent media, such as a backup server, and is always at the level of the last backup of the server, with a list of changes.

- *Continuous backup,* where data on the system is immediately written to backup media.

With a digital image archive, two methods of backup are usually required; one for the server (including the archive database, demographics, etc.) and one for the actual image data. The server backup can adopt any of the strategies above, but the image data is nearly always backed up to a continuous archive.

A typical mid-sized system would therefore have a daily incremental backup of the server, probably on to tape or DVD, and continuous backup of the images as they are acquired, stored to the RAID. It is prudent for the backup to be at a different physical location to the RAID so that if there were a fire, for instance, the system could be rebuilt.

A third party with a data vault may provide offsite storage; to the user this would appear as any other archive, however it could actually be anywhere in the world. This type of system does have limitations of speed of access as the Internet is used to transfer the data, and there may be issues of data protection and security.

Example Systems

The following diagrams bring together schematically the elements described above into simple solutions for two typical scenarios. The first scenario is where a single digital device, such as an intraoral detector, is installed. The second is where there are multiple devices (e.g. several intraoral and one panoramic unit), with a single workstation remote from the acquisition devices. The multi-modality model could also readily be scaled up for larger institutions, with multiple departments, modalities and devices and several workstations.

Single-modality System *(Fig 8-11)*
This type of system may be supplied as a bespoke solution from the modality manufacturer. It has no need to connect to other devices and does not need to archive onto backup media or to print. Images are directly reported from the computer display. There is no need for DICOM, unless a DICOM printer is used or images need to be transferred to other sites; nor is there a need for HL7 compatibility as patient data is entered for each new patient directly and stored in the on-board database. This type of system in its simplest form is vulnerable to SPFs and theft. It is advised that a full-system

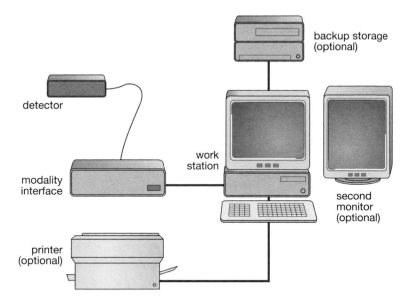

Fig 8-11 Simple single-device system.

backup methodology is used (see above) and that a RAID is installed at a minimum of RAID 1. It is important that the database is also backed up. If the system is likely to expand then DICOM Store is required:

DICOM SOP:Store:SCU:(DICOM Object type).
DICOM SOP:Modality Worklist:SCP:(DICOM Object type).
DICOM SOP:Print:SCU:(DICOM Object type).

Multi-modality System (Fig 8-12)
This type of system may also be supplied as a bespoke solution from a modality manufacturer, however it is likely that it will be configured from many different manufacturers' products, either by a PACS provider or by a local IT team. Each modality is effectively a mirror of the set-up for a single-modality system; indeed, even keeping limited local storage is still desirable in case there are network or PACS failures. However, backup will be handled centrally, as will print and interface functions. DICOM functions such as Print are now required if a DICOM printer is centrally connected. There is also now a need for HL7 compatibility as patient data will come from the HIS or from the radiology or practice management software, where the patient has been booked onto the system at reception.

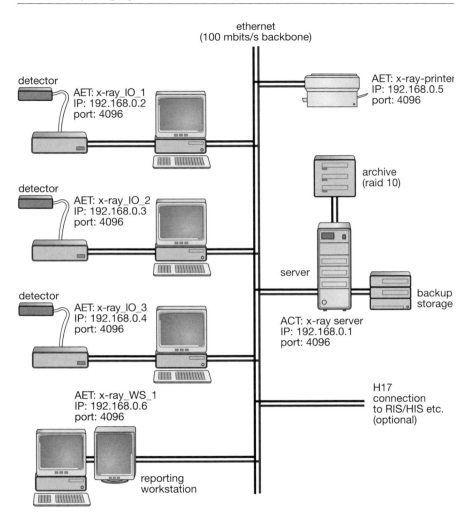

Fig 8-12 Multiple devices and single workstation.

Further Reading

Aldrich JE, Rutledge JD. Assessment of PACS display systems. J Digit Imaging 2005;18(4):287–295.

Brettle DS. Commentary: Soft copy display requirements for hospital wide image viewing. Br J Radiol 2007 (in press).

Deutsches Instituit für Normung. DIN EN 60529, Degrees of Protection Provided by Enclosures (IP code). DIN, 2000.

Doyle AJ, Le Fevre J, Anderson JD. Personal computer versus workstation display: observer performance in detection of wrist fractures on digital radiographs. Radiology 2005;237(3):872-877.

Fuchsjager MH, Schaefer-Prokop CM, Eisenhuber E, et al., Impact of ambient light and window settings on the detectability of catheters on soft-copy display of chest radiographs at bedside. AJR Am J Roentgenol 2003;181(5):1415-1421.

Haak R, Wicht MJ, Hellmich M, Nowak G, Noack MJ. Influence of room lighting on grey-scale perception with a CRT and a TFT monitor display. Dentomaxillofac Radiol 2002;31(3):193-197.

Institute of Physics and Engineering in Medicine. Recommended Standards for the Routine Performance Testing of Diagnostic X-ray Imaging Systems. IPEM Report 91. York: IPEM, 2005, p. 112.

International Electrotechnical Commission. Medical Electrical Equipment - Part 1: General requirements for basic safety and essential performance. In: IEC 60601-1. IEC, 2005.

Krupinski EA, Johnson J, Roehrig H, et al. Use of a human visual system model to predict observer performance with CRT vs LCD display of images. J Digit Imaging 2004;17(4):258-263.

Medicines and Healthcare Products Regulatory Agency. PACSNet. Beginners Guide to Networks: Part I & II. MHRA Report 03053, 2003. (www.pasa.doh.gov.uk/evaluation/publications/)

Medicines and Healthcare Products Regulatory Agency. Display Image Quality. MHRA, 2004.

Oosterwijk H. DICOM Basics. 2nd edn. 2002, OTech Inc.

Samei E. AAPM/RSNA physics tutorial for residents: technological and psychophysical considerations for digital mammographic displays. Radiographics 2005;25(2):491-501.

Samei E, Badano A, Chakraborty D, et al. Assessment of display performance for medical imaging systems: executive summary of AAPM TG18 report. Med Phys 2005;32(4):1205-1225.

Samei E. et al. Assessment of Display Performance for Medical Imaging Systems, Medical Physics Publishing. Report of the American Association of Physicists in Medicine (AAPM) Task Group 18. Madison, WI, 2005.

137

Saunders RS Jr, Samei E. Resolution and noise measurements of five CRT and LCD medical displays. Med Phys 2006;33(2):308-319.

Society of Motion Pictures and Television Engineers. RP 133: Specifications for medical diagnostic imaging test pattern for television monitors and hard-copy recording cameras. New York: SMPTE, 1991, p. 6.

Chapter 9

Implant Imaging

Aim

Implantology is a major growth area in dentistry and uses a greater range of imaging techniques than other aspects of the profession. The aim of this chapter is to provide information about implant imaging.

Outcome

After reading this chapter, the reader should be able to:
- give the indications for imaging in implantology
- list the advantages and disadvantages of the imaging techniques used in implant imaging
- state the doses of the common radiographic techniques used in implantology
- appreciate the concept of tomography and be familiar with the tomographic techniques that may be used in implantology.

Indications for Imaging

Imaging is essential in implantology. It is required at the following stages:
- preoperative
- intraoperative
- post-operative.

Table 9-1 summarises the indications for imaging and suggests appropriate views at these stages.

Imaging Techniques

The following investigations are frequently used in implant imaging:
- periapical radiographs
- occlusal radiographs (mandible)
- dental panoramic tomographs
- lateral cephalometric views
- cross-sectional imaging (tomography and computed tomography).

Table 9-1 **Indications for imaging during implantology, and the appropriate views at each stage** (continued over page)

Stage	Indication	Appropriate radiographic views	Additional notes
Pre-operative	• To establish the optimum position for the proposed implants • To identify important anatomical structures within the jaws, so they can be avoided during surgery • To assess the morphology of the bone, since a minimum height, width and volume of bone is required • To identify undercuts within the bone • To examine the quality of the bone, since implants placed in poor quality bone are more likely to fail • To exclude the presence of occult disease	• Periapical radiograph • Dental panoramic tomograph • Occlusal radiograph (mandible) • Lateral cephalometric radiograph • Cross-sectional imaging	• Radiographs need to be geometrically accurate • In *uncomplicated* single implant cases, cross-sectional imaging not normally necessary
Intra-operative	• In difficult cases to facilitate precise positioning of the implant	• Periapical radiograph	• Radiographs need to be geometrically accurate • Digital radiography useful as images are displayed more quickly than with conventional radiography

Table 9-1 **Indications for imaging during implantology, and the appropriate views at each stage** (continued)

Stage	Indication	Appropriate radiographic views	Additional notes
Post-operative	• To assess osseointegration • To assess long-term bony support	• Periapical radiograph • Dental panoramic tomograph • Rarely other specialised techniques	• Radiography essential if symptomatic • Radiographs need to be geometrically accurate so that the threads on the fixtures can be visualised • Digital subtraction radiography may be used to assess osseointegration • Rate of vertical bone loss should be less than 0.2 mm annually following the first year of placement • Radiographic review every 1–3 years until there is no evidence of continued bone loss • Computed tomography should not normally be used as the fixtures can cause significant artefacts

The advantages and disadvantages of these techniques are shown in Table 9-2 (pages 143 and 144) and typical doses are shown in Table 9-3 (page 146).

Cross-sectional Imaging

Concept of Tomography

With conventional radiography, structures that lie along the same path as the emerging x-ray beam are superimposed on each other in the final image. As a result, overlying tissues may obscure those structures under investigation. Tomographic techniques can be used to produce a "slice", or focal layer, to allow the required structures to be seen.

The simplest form of tomography is linear tomography. The x-ray tube and cassette are linked together and move in opposite directions about a fulcrum. A broad x-ray beam is used and the radiographic exposure is continuous throughout the movement. Three points, A, B and C, are shown in Fig 9-1 (page 145). If a conventional radiograph is taken, these objects become superimposed and little information can be gained. In this example, we shall assume information is required about point B, so this point is made the fulcrum of the movement.

- At the start of the movement, the centre of the beam passes through point B and is projected onto the centre of the film.
- During the movement, the x-ray tube and the film are moving at the same speed but in opposite directions. Point B is therefore always projected onto the centre of the film and so is in focus.
- All structures in the plane parallel to the x-ray source passing through point B will also be in focus, producing a "slice" or focal layer.
- A structure at point A is initially projected onto the right side of the film, but at the end of the movement is projected onto the left side, and so becomes blurred.
- A structure at point C at the start is projected onto the left side of the film, but at the end of the movement is projected onto the right side, so also becomes blurred.
- All the structures lying outside the focal plane are thus intentionally blurred out. The further the structures are from the focal plane, the more blurred they become.
- The blurring on the image is always in the same direction as the movement, and may produce linear "streaking artefacts".

An example of a linear tomograph is shown in Fig 9-2 (page 145).

142

Table 9-2 **Advantages and disadvantages of the various radiographic techniques used in implantology**

(continued over page).

(Adapted from *Radiation Protection 136: European Guidelines on Radiation Protection in Dental Radiology: the safe use of radiographs in dental practice*)

Technique	Advantages	Disadvantages
Periapical radiography	• Excellent resolution • Inexpensive • Low dose • Gives a vertical and horizontal measurement of bone available • Reproducible images obtained if the paralleling technique is used	• Difficult to obtain reproducible images in edentulous patients • No cross-sectional information
Occlusal radiography	• Excellent resolution • Inexpensive • Low dose • Shows width of the mandible • May show the course of the inferior dental canal and mental foramen • May be used as a planning view in tomography	• No cross-sectional information • Only helpful in the mandible
Dental panoramic tomography	• Low cost • Relatively low dose • Whole of mandible/maxilla can be seen on one film • Gives a vertical and horizontal measurement of bone available	• Low resolution • No cross-sectional information • High inherent magnification • Magnification in vertical and horizontal planes not necessarily equal • Technique errors can lead to further geometric distortion
Lateral cephalo-metric radiography	• Reproducible and accurate technique • Provides some cross-sectional information on the midline structures of the jaws	• Low resolution • Because of superimposition, can only be used to assess the anterior region • Cephalometric equipment not necessarily available to the general dental practitioner

Table 9-2 **Advantages and disadvantages of radiographic techniques** (cont).

Technique	Advantages	Disadvantages
Cross-sectional tomography (spiral/ hypocy-cloidal)	• Provides cross-sectional information • Accurate measurements • Imaging limited to sites of interest	• Long acquisition time • Tomographic blur present on image • Technically difficult to perform • Tomographic blurring can make interpretation difficult • Limited availability • Relatively high dose • Moderately expensive • Bone density measurements not possible
Computed tomography (conventional)	• Provides cross-sectional information • Accurate • Short acquisition time • No superimposed tomographic blurring • Multiplanar views and 3-D reconstruction possible • Uniform magnification • Bone density measurements possible	• High dose • Imaging of entire jaw rather than site of interest • Amalgam can cause significant artefacts on image • Limited availability • Expensive
Cone beam computed tomography	• Provides cross-sectional information • Accurate • Short acquisition time • No superimposed tomographic blurring • Multiplanar views and 3-D reconstruction possible • Uniform magnification • Technically straightforward to perform • Lower dose than conventional CT • PC based software	• Imaging of entire jaw rather than site of interest • Limited availability • Relatively expensive • Amalgam can cause artefacts on image • Limited bone density information provided
Magnetic resonance imaging	• No radiation dose • Provides cross-sectional information • Measurements accurate • No amalgam artefacts • Excellent contrast resolution	• No specific software programmes available to help with planning • Difficult to interpret for the inexperienced • Very limited availability • Expensive

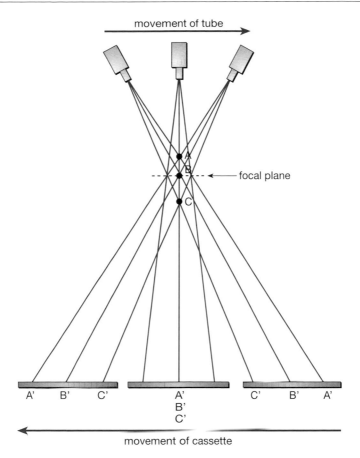

movement of tube →

●A
●B ←— focal plane
●C

A'   B'   C'   A'   C'   B'   A'
                      B'
                      C'

← movement of cassette

Fig 9-1 Diagram showing the principle of linear tomography. Point B is projected (B') onto the same part of the film at all times and will therefore be in focus. Some panoramic machines employ this method of tomography to produce cross-sectional images of the jaws. A', B' and C' = images of points A, B and C respectively.

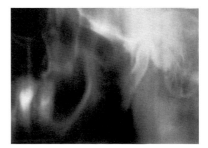

Fig 9-2 Example of a linear tomograph demonstrating the left temporomandibular joint. The movement of the tube and cassette in this case are in a vertical direction. Note that the structures outside the focal layer are blurred out and produce vertical linear "streaking" artefacts.

145

Table 9-3 **Typical effective doses from common radiographic investigations used in implantology**

★Estimate not based on published figures ★★Wide variation in dose partly due to differences in scanning parameters utilised. Using modern scanning protocols, the expected doses would be at the lower end of this range.

Imaging technique	Effective dose μSv	Equivalent natural background radiation dose in the UK
Periapical radiograph	1–8	4–32 hours
Lower occlusal radiograph★	2–8	8–32 hours
Dental panoramic tomograph (if salivary glands included in the calculations)	16–26	2.6–4.3 days
Cephalometric lateral skull	3–5	12–20 hours
Cross-sectional slice on a panoramic machine (molar region)	9	36 hours
Single cross-sectional slice using spiral tomography	1–30	4 hours–5 days
CT mandible★★	480–3324	80 days–1.5 years
CT maxilla★★	240–1200	40 days–6.7 months
Cone beam CT mandible (if salivary glands included in the calculations)	75	12.5 days
Cone beam CT maxilla (if salivary glands included in the calculations)	42	7 days

Cross-sectional Imaging in Implantology

The techniques that may be used in implantology include:

- linear tomography and rotational narrow-beam tomography
- complex motion tomography
- computed tomography (CT)
- cone beam computed tomography (CBCT)
- magnetic resonance imaging (MRI).

Linear Tomography and Rotational Narrow–beam Tomography

Most panoramic units are available with an optional cross–sectional imaging facility, which makes them attractive to the general dental practitioner. These programmes may be based on the concept of conventional linear tomography or rotational narrow-beam tomography.

- *Conventional linear tomography.* An example of a conventional linear tomography unit is the OP100 (Instrumentarium Dental, Tuusula, Finland). The x-ray tube and film cassette move about a fulcrum, which coincides with the focal layer. This uses the same tomographic movement as shown in Fig 9-1.

- *Rotational narrow-beam tomography.* The Planmeca 2002CC transversal slicing system (Planmeca Oy, Helsinki, Finland) provides rotational narrow-beam tomography. The image is formed in a similar fashion to a dental panoramic tomograph, but a single centre of rotation is used (Fig 9-3). A curved focal layer is created because the narrow beam moves through the region of interest at the same speed as the film cassette is moving behind the slit in the cassette holder.

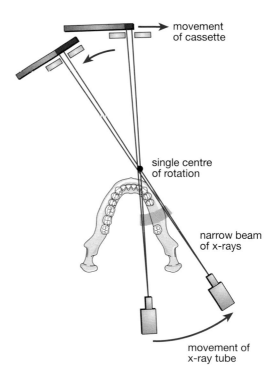

movement
of cassette

single centre
of rotation

narrow beam
of x-rays

movement of
x-ray tube

Fig 9-3 Diagram showing the principle of rotational narrow-beam tomography. This technique produces a curved focal layer of the jaw. (Courtesy of Instrumentarium Dental).

147

Practical procedure
Once the appropriate programme is chosen and the exposure factors are set, the patient is positioned within the machine. The patient is positioned as they would be for a panoramic image, except that the chin may be raised so that the lower border of the mandible is parallel to the floor (Fig 9-4).

With some machines a silicone impression of the dental arch is required to position the patient correctly. The impression, attached to a biteplate, is secured to the panoramic unit. Two positioning lights are used to ensure the area of interest is coincident with the cross-sectional layer. The patient then places the teeth back into the impression and the radiographic exposure is made. Several exposures may be carried out on one film, and so the patient must be instructed to keep still for a relatively long period of time.

On most machines the slice thickness can be altered. The cross-sectional angle is, however, often preset and cannot be altered. Some systems only permit tomography of the posterior part of the arch, while other machines can produce slices parallel to the dental arch (sagittal slices).

Image quality
Magnification of the cross-sectional image is often greater than for panoramic radiographs, making direct comparison between images difficult. The magnification factor is generally x1.5, whereas the magnification for the panoramic image is about x1.2.

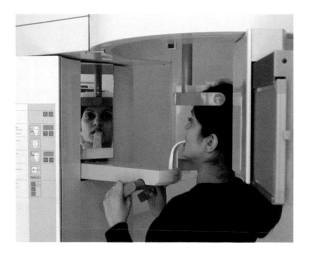

Fig 9-4 Patient positioned in a panoramic machine for cross-sectional imaging. Note that in this case the patient is positioned so that the lower border of the mandible is horizontal.

There can be problems with uneven magnification in the horizontal and vertical planes with the systems based on rotational narrow-beam tomography. Some researchers have found, using the slicing systems on panoramic machines, that the slice thickness is too thick to allow accurate assessment of the bone. Others, though, have found that these images can be used to assess vertical distances. Little research has been carried out to establish whether measurements in the horizontal plane are accurate or if the morphology of the bone is correctly represented. A typical set of images is shown in Fig 9-5.

Complex Motion Tomography
With linear tomography, overlying blurred shadows can mask the image layer, making interpretation difficult. More complicated movements of the x-ray tube and film cassette produce more effective blurring of the adjacent structures and reduce artefacts. These complex motions include spiral and hypocycloidal tomography. As well as improving image quality, the complex movements also make it possible to produce thinner cross-sections.
• Spiral tomography. Examples of units employing spiral tomography are the Scanora and the Cranex Tome (Soredex, Tuusula, Finland)
• Hypocycloidal tomography. The Panorex CMT (Imaging Sciences International, Hatfield, PA, USA) uses hypocycloidal tomography.

The Scanora and Panorex CMT are dedicated machines for imaging the maxillofacial complex. These machines are normally found in the hospital setting or occasionally in specialist radiographic practice. The Cranex Tome, however, is a panoramic machine appropriate for general dental practice.

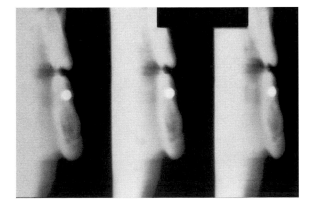

Fig 9-5 A typical set of cross-sectional images of the left mandible produced on a panoramic machine. (Courtesy of Mrs JE Brown).

Practical procedure
With the Scanora system, an impression of the teeth and alveolus may be required to construct an acrylic radiographic stent. The stent contains radiopaque markers made from either gutta-percha or metal placed at the proposed sites of the implants (Fig 9-6). The patient wears the stent throughout the examination. Initially, a panoramic radiograph is obtained so that the regions of interest can be identified.

• *Region selection.* The panoramic radiograph is placed on a dedicated x-ray viewing box that has a numbered scale marked along the edge. The cursor on the viewing box is adjusted to lie over the area proposed for implants. The number on the scale corresponds to the area of the jaw to be imaged (Fig 9-7).

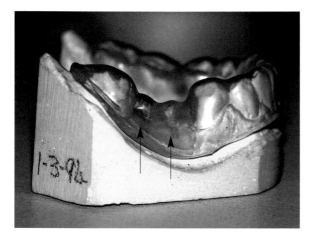

Fig 9-6 Radiographic stent constructed of soft acrylic. Radiopaque markers (arrowed) have been placed in the stent.

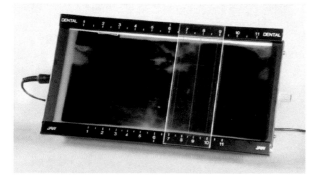

Fig 9-7 Panoramic film on dedicated implant planning viewing box. The sliding cursor and horizontal scale on the box are used to select the region of interest. (Courtesy of Mr E Whaites).

- *Cross-section selection.* An acetate sheet containing a printed outline of an average jaw and choice of cross-sections is placed over the model and a suitable cross-section selected. If a model is not available, or the ridge form is not sufficiently well reproduced, then a lower occlusal radiograph may be used for this purpose.
- *Slice-thickness selection.* A slice thickness of 2 mm, 4 mm or 8 mm can be chosen. For the posterior region, 4 mm is normally preferred. In contrast, 2 mm tends to be selected for the anterior region.

The combination of region, cross-section angle and slice-thickness corresponds to a three-digit code, which is programmed into the control panel. The exposure factors vary between 60 and 66 kV and 1.6 and 6.4 mA, depending upon region and patient size. The patient is positioned accurately in the machine using laser positioning guides and the tomograms are obtained (Fig 9-8). A single slice can take up to 90 seconds. It is therefore important that the patient is able to keep still throughout the exposure. The radiopaque markers in the stent allow the site of the cross-section to be identified. Examples of images obtained using spiral tomography are shown in Fig 9-9.

The technique is operator sensitive, and a great deal of expertise is required to use the machine successfully. This system is particularly useful if cross-sectional information is required for a single site. The process is time consuming, so should not be considered for imaging multiple sites, or for elderly or frail patients who might find it difficult to remain still for long periods of time. In addition, the dose is dependent upon the number of sites being imaged. Therefore, if multiple sites are required, other techniques may give the required information at a lower dose.

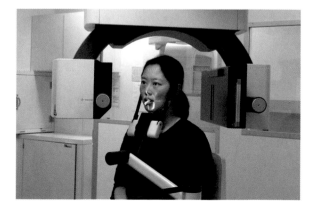

Fig 9-8 Patient seated in the Scanora unit, a machine that employs spiral tomography. The laser markers are used to position the patient correctly.

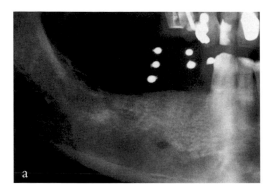

Fig 9-9 Examples of cross-sectional images produced by spiral tomography on the Scanora unit; a) cropped panoramic radiograph showing radiographic markers; b) cross-sectional images.

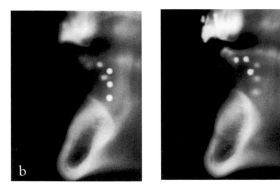

Image quality

Because complex motion is employed, the image quality is better than in linear tomography. There is always some inherent blurring present on the images, but it has been shown to be an accurate technique for assessing bone height and width and for identifying structures such as the inferior dental canal. The cross-sectional images and the panoramic images are magnified by the same factor (x1.7), so direct comparison between images is possible. However, interpretation of the images requires training, and no information is provided on bone density.

Computed Tomography

A CT scanner consists of a table and a gantry that contains an x-ray source and detectors. The patient lies on the table, which is moved through an aperture in the gantry while a narrow fan-shaped x-ray beam rotates about the patient. The attenuated x-ray beam is detected by an array of detectors, and the resultant signal is used to construct a cross-sectional slice of the region.

Several generations of CT scanner exist. The common types in use today are third-generation scanners, fourth-generation scanners and spiral scanners.

Third-generation scanners
These scanners (Fig 9-10):
- use a narrow fan-shaped x-ray beam
- typically have ionisation chamber type detectors
- generally have fewer detectors (several hundred) than fourth-generation machines
- have detectors arranged in a curvilinear fashion, with the x-ray source aligned with the detectors
- involve the x-ray source and the detectors rotating through 360° around the patient.

Fourth-generation scanners
These scanners (Fig 9-11):
- use a narrow fan-shaped x-ray beam
- typically have solid-state detectors
- generally have more detectors (up to 2000) than third-generation machines
- have detectors arranged in a complete ring
- involve the x-ray source rotating through 360° around the patient whilst the detectors remain stationary.

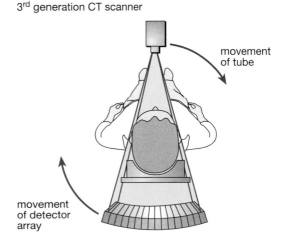

3rd generation CT scanner

movement of tube

movement of detector array

Fig 9-10 Diagram showing the arrangement of the detectors and the x-ray tube in a third-generation CT scanner.

4th generation
CT scanner

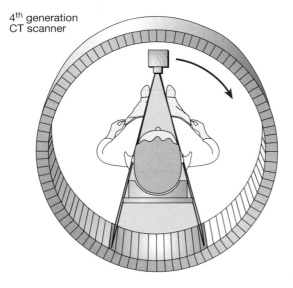

Fig 9-11 Diagram showing the arrangement of the detectors and x-ray tube in a fourth-generation CT scanner.

Spiral scanners

Some modern CT scanners use "slip ring" technology to supply the power to the x-ray tube. Since there are no cables hindering the movement of the x-ray source, continuous rotation is possible. This permits spiral or helical scanning. With these systems the table moves at a uniform speed through the gantry aperture, whilst the tube and detectors move continuously around the patient. A coil-shaped data set is collected, from which reconstruction into the required plane is performed.

Spiral scanning has many technical advantages. For implant imaging these include:
- faster scan times
- fewer motion artefacts due to swallowing
- improved reformatting into other planes, a feature particularly useful with implant imaging.

Detectors used in CT scanners

The detectors in CT scanners are arranged in either a circular or curvilinear array and may be of two types:
- *Solid-state detectors.* These are composed of crystals that fluoresce when irradiated. The light emitted is detected and amplified by a photomultiplier tube to produce a voltage.

154

- *Ionisation chambers.* These are gas-filled chambers separated by tungsten electrodes. When irradiated the gas is ionised and the ions are attracted to the electrodes, producing a current.

Whichever type of detector is used, the resultant signal is proportional to the number of incoming x-ray photons incident on the detector.

Image construction
A matrix of 512 x 512 voxels (volume elements) is allocated to each slice. The production of a cross-sectional image through an arm is illustrated in Fig 9-12. If a 5 mm slice were obtained, then each voxel would typically measure 1 mm x 1 mm x 5 mm, the width of the voxel being equivalent to the slice thickness. The computer calculates the amount of attenuation of the beam at each voxel. Complicated algorithms are used to reconstruct the image as a matrix of 512 x 512 pixels (picture elements). Each pixel is assigned a number corresponding to the amount of attenuation in each voxel. These numbers are known as CT or Hounsfield numbers.

Water has a CT number of 0, air -1000 and bone +1000. Bone, and in particular cortical bone, can be very dense and may be assigned a much higher number (up to +3000). Typical CT numbers are shown in Table 9-4, page 157. These numbers correspond to a shade of grey on the image.

As shown in Table 9-4, the range of CT numbers is wide. As the visual apparatus cannot distinguish this range of grey shades, the image is altered to display the tissue densities of the particular structures under investigation. This is achieved by altering the "window width" and "window level".

The window width is the range of CT numbers over which the grey range is displayed. The window level is the centre of this range. Tissues outside of this range are displayed either black or white (Fig 9-13). The window level and width are normally selected from the imaging protocols. These windows are sometimes loosely referred to as "soft tissue" or "bony" windows. An example of the same data displayed on either soft tissue and bony windows is shown in Fig 9-14.

Practical procedure
Most CT scans are performed axially, which is comfortable for the patient. The data is then reformatted to produce cross-sections in the required plane. There are many CT software programmes available for implant planning.

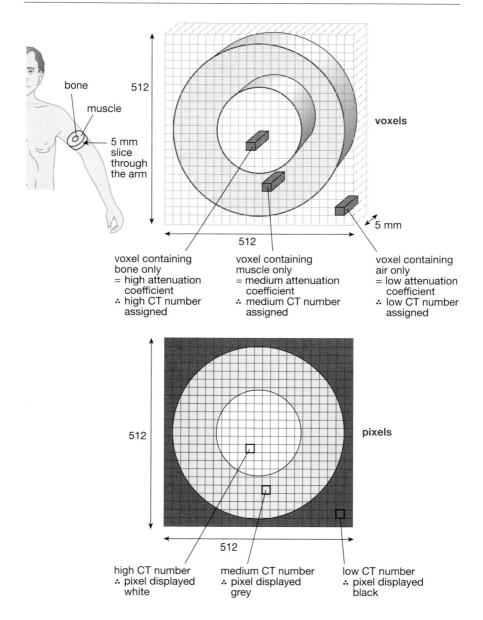

Fig 9-12 Diagram showing how a CT image is constructed. In this example, a 5 mm slice through the arm is being produced, and each voxel is 1 x 1 x 5 mm. The computer calculates the amount of attenuation of the beam at each voxel. This is then assigned a CT number, and ultimately displayed as a shade of grey on a matrix size of 512 x 512.

Table 9-4 **Typical CT numbers**

Material	CT number	Shade of grey
bone	+ 1000	white
muscle	+ 30–60	
water	0	mid-grey
fat	– 100	
air	– 1000	black

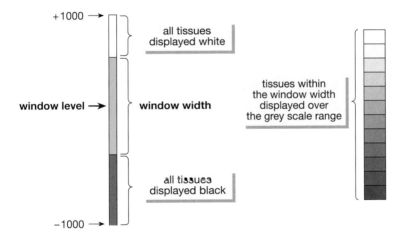

Fig 9-13 The window width is the range of CT numbers over which the greyscale is displayed, and the window level is the centre of this range. Appropriate window width and level are chosen depending upon the tissues under investigation.

One such programme is DentaScan (GE Medical Systems, Milwaukee, USA). The patient lies supine on the table and the head positioned so the lower border of the mandible is parallel to the scan plane (for imaging the mandible) or the hard palate is parallel to the scan plane (for imaging the maxilla) (Fig 9-15). The head is immobilised and a "scout view" is obtained of the jaw. The scout view is a lateral view of the jaws, and is used to select

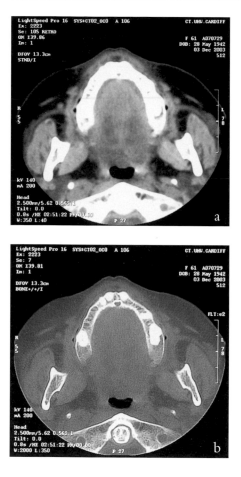

Fig 9-14 An example of how changing the window level and width enables both the soft tissues and hard tissues to be displayed correctly; a) displayed on soft tissue windows; b) displayed on bony windows.

the start and finish positions of the scan and to make sure that the jaw is parallel to the scan plane.

Scanning is normally performed using a kilovoltage of around 140 kV and a current setting of 60 mA. If helical scanning is used, each rotation takes 1 second, so a scan of the jaw can take as little as 12 seconds. The width level applied is typically 350 and the window width 2000.

Initially, the axial slices are displayed on the screen. By selecting multiple points on one of the images, the software programme links up the points to produce a curve through the jaw. Images can then be reconstructed

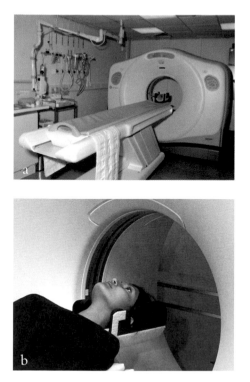

Fig 9-15 a) An example of a CT scanner; b) The patient has been positioned in the scanner to examine the maxilla.

either parallel to this curve to produce panoramic type images or perpendicular to this curve to produce cross-sectional images (Fig 9-16). The images have a millimetre scale adjacent to the image to facilitate measurements.

There are software programmes that can be used to simulate the proposed implant placement prior to surgery. This allows the correct size and orientation of the implant fixtures to be determined. This information may be used to construct acrylic drill guides with drill holes at the proposed implant sites. In this way the implants can be placed at exactly the same site and angulation as previously planned on the computer simulation.

Image quality
CT is generally regarded as the most accurate method of imaging the jaws for implant assessment. Measurements of bone height are very accurate, and a precise assessment can be made of the ridge morphology. There is no

159

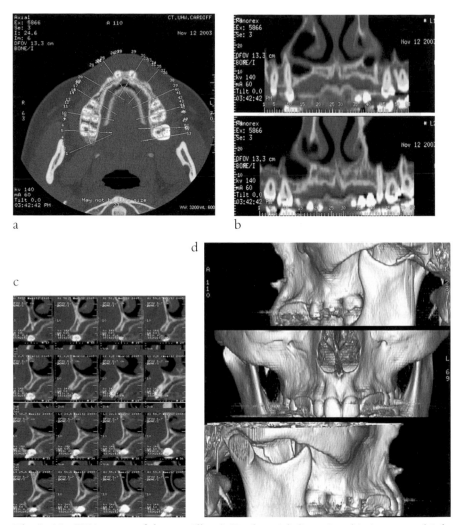

Fig 9-16 CT images of the maxilla; a) Single axial slice. On this image multiple points have been selected by the operator along the central part of the alveolar ridge. The computer programme joins these points together to produce a curve through the jaw; b) Reconstructed images parallel to the curve, producing panoramic type image; c) Reconstructed images perpendicular to the curve, producing cross-sectional images. These images are the most useful when assessing the bone for the suitability for implant placement; d) Three-dimensional reconstruction of the maxilla.

overlying blur in the images. The contrast resolution is high and allows differentiation of structures with only small differences in density. If required, the bone density can be measured. Three-dimensional reconstructions can be performed, although these are not particularly useful in planning surgery. The main drawback to using CT is the high dose.

Cone Beam Computed Tomography (CBCT)

There are CT scanners available that are dedicated for use in the maxillofacial region. These units have been referred to as low-dose CT scanners and use a simpler technology than the systems described above. In these systems, the detector is flat, comprising either an image intensifier coupled to a CCD or a silicone panel. A cone-shaped x-ray beam is generated, rather than a fan-

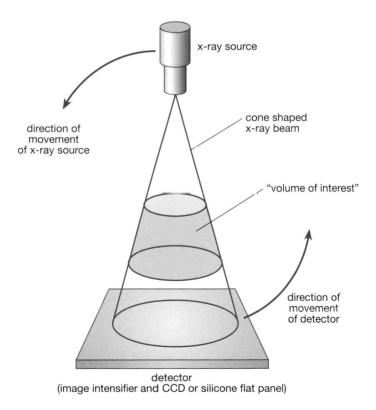

x-ray source

direction of
movement
of x-ray source

cone shaped
x-ray beam

"volume of interest"

direction of
movement
of detector

detector
(image intensifier and CCD or silicone flat panel)

Fig 9-17 Diagram showing the principle of CBCT. The x-ray source produces a cone-shaped x-ray beam that acquires a volume of the region of interest in a single rotation.

shaped beam (Fig 9-17). This allows the jaws to be imaged in a single rotation, without the need for a moving table. The x-ray field may be collimated to include the jaw of interest only. Scanning is quick, with a scan time of 10–40 seconds. The high contrast resolution is good, allowing excellent depiction of bony detail, although soft tissue contrast is poor. Accurate assessments of bone height, width and morphology can be made. The effective dose using these systems is typically much less than that for conventional and spiral CT, although the dose is dependent on the volume of tissue irradiated. There are several commercial systems on the market, including the Newtom 9000 (NIM s.r.l., Verona, Italy) (Fig 9-18a) and the i-CAT (Imaging Sciences International, Hatfield, PA, USA) (Fig 9-18b).

Although the machines are expensive, they are significantly cheaper than a conventional CT scanner. This makes them suitable for dental hospitals or specialist dental practices. Examples of images obtained by this method are shown in Fig 9-19.

Magnetic Resonance Imaging

MRI has been suggested as an alternative to CT because cross-sectional images are produced without using ionising radiation. It has been shown to be an effective imaging modality in the assessment of the jaws for implant planning. However, all MRI scanners are currently hospital based and scanning is expensive. Interpretation of the scans can be difficult for those unfamiliar with the modality, because cortical bone is shown black (as opposed to white on a CT scan) and the medullary bone is white/grey.

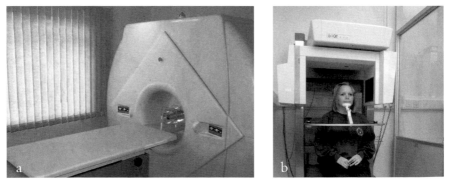

Fig 9-18 Examples of CBCT Scanners; a) the Newtom 9000 (courtesy of Dr Colin Cook); b) the i-CAT.

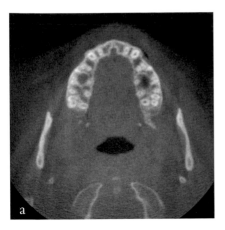

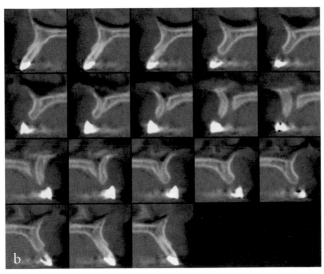

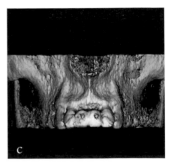

Fig 9-19 Examples of images produced on a CBCT scanner; a) single axial image of the maxilla; b) cross-sectional images of the anterior region; c) three-dimensional reconstruction of the maxilla. (Courtesy of Dr Colin Cook).

163

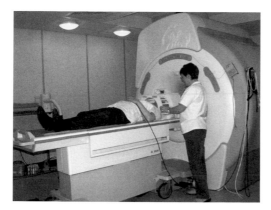

Fig 9-20 An example of an MRI scanner. The patient is being prepared for a scan of the jaws. Note how close the detectors are to the head. This can sometimes cause problems if the patient is claustrophobic. (Courtesy of Dr Crawford Gray).

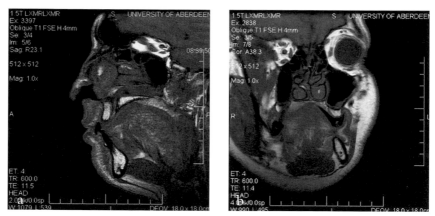

Fig 9-21 Cross-sectional images produced on an MRI scanner. Note that in both images the cortical bone is black (no signal) and the medullary bone is bright (high signal); a) midline; b) left posterior mandible. (Courtesy of Dr Crawford Gray).

Currently, there is a lack of dedicated software programmes for implant planning. For these reasons, this imaging modality is not widely used at the present time, but it is likely to become more popular in the future. An MRI scanner and typical images are shown in Figs 9-20 and 9-21.

Indications for Cross-sectional Imaging
There is little evidence-based guidance on the indications for cross-sectional imaging in implantology. The American Academy of Oral and Maxillofacial Radiology recommends that the evaluation of any potential implant site

includes cross-sectional imaging. The Academy recommends spiral tomography or hypocycloidal tomography if there are seven or fewer implant sites and computed tomography if there are more than seven implant sites.

The European Association for Osseointegration is more selective in its recommendations for cross-sectional imaging. The Association recommends that if clinical and radiographic examination (intraoral or panoramic radiography) shows sufficient bone to place implants, then further cross-sectional imaging is seldom necessary. Its recommendations for cross-sectional imaging of the jaws include when:

- the implant site is close to inferior dental canal or incisive canal
- there is extreme ridge atrophy
- bone augmentation or grafting is being considered
- a fixed prosthesis is being planned and information is required to produce optimal loading of the implant
- there is clinical doubt about the shape of the alveolar ridge
- maxillary sinus descends close to the proposed implant site.

Key Points

- Imaging may be required at the preoperative planning, intraoperative and post-operative stages.
- Cross-sectional imaging is required in planning complicated implant cases.
- The choice of cross-sectional modality is determined by several factors, including number of proposed implant sites, image quality, patient dose and the availability of equipment.

Further Reading

Carlton RR, Adler AM. Tomography. In: Carlton RR, Adler AM (eds). Principles of Radiographic Imaging; an art and a science. 3rd edn. Albany, NY: Delmar, 2001.

Carlton RR, Adler AM. Computed tomography. In: Carlton RR, Adler AM (eds). Principles of Radiographic Imaging; an art and a science. 3rd edn. Albany, NY: Delmar, 2001.

European Commission. Radiation Protection 136. European Guidelines on Radiation Protection in Dental Radiology. The safe use of radiographs in dental practice. EC, 2004.

Harris D, Buser D, Dula K, et al. E.A.O. Guidelines for the use of diagnostic imaging in implant dentistry. Clin Oral Implan Res 2002;13:566-570.

Tyndall D, Brooks S. Selection criteria for dental implant site imaging: A position paper of the American Academy of Oral and Maxillofacial Radiology. Oral Surg Oral Med Oral Pathol Oral Radiol Endod 2000;89:630–637.

Index

Quintessentials for General Dental Practitioners Series

in 50 volumes

Editor-in-Chief: Professor Nairn H F Wilson

The Quintessentials for General Dental Practitioners Series covers basic principles and key issues in all aspects of modern dental medicine. Each book can be read as a stand-alone volume or in conjunction with other books in the series.

Publication date,
approximately

Clinical Practice, Editor: Nairn Wilson

Culturally Sensitive Oral Healthcare	available
Dental Erosion	available
Special Care Dentistry	available
Evidence Based Dentistry	Autumn 2007
Infection Control for the Dental Team	Winter 2007
Therapeutics and Medical Emergencies in the Everyday Clinical Practice of Dentistry	Winter 2007

Oral Surgery and Oral Medicine, Editor: John G Meechan

Practical Dental Local Anaesthesia	available
Practical Oral Medicine	available
Practical Conscious Sedation	available
Minor Oral Surgery in Dental Practice	available

Imaging, Editor: Keith Horner

Interpreting Dental Radiographs	available
Panoramic Radiology	available
21st Century Dental Imaging	available

Periodontology, Editor: Iain L C Chapple

Understanding Periodontal Diseases: Assessment and Diagnostic Procedures in Practice	available
Decision-Making for the Periodontal Team	available
Successful Periodontal Therapy – A Non-Surgical Approach	available
Periodontal Management of Children, Adolescents and Young Adults	available
Periodontal Medicine: A Window on the Body	available
Contemporary Periodontal Surgery – An Illustrated Guide to the Art Behind the Science	Autumn 2007

Endodontics, Editor: John M Whitworth

Rational Root Canal Treatment in Practice	available
Managing Endodontic Failure in Practice	available
Adhesive Restoration of Endodontically Treated Teeth	available

Prosthodontics, Editor: P Finbarr Allen

Teeth for Life for Older Adults	available
Complete Dentures – from Planning to Problem Solving	available
Removable Partial Dentures	available
Fixed Prosthodontics in Dental Practice	available
Occlusion: A Theoretical and Team Approach	Autumn 2007
Managing Orofacial Pain in Practice	Winter 2007

Operative Dentistry, Editor: Paul A Brunton

Decision-Making in Operative Dentistry	available
Aesthetic Dentistry	available
Communicating in Dental Practice	available
Indirect Restorations	available
Dental Bleaching	available
Choosing and Using Dental Materials	Autumn 2007
Composite Restorations in Posterior Teeth	Winter 2007

Paediatric Dentistry/Orthodontics, Editor: Marie Therese Hosey

Child Taming: How to Manage Children in Dental Practice	available
Paediatric Cariology	available
Treatment Planning for the Developing Dentition	available
Managing Dental Trauma in Practice	available

General Dentistry and Practice Management, Editor: Raj Rattan

The Business of Dentistry	available
Risk Management in General Dental Practice	available
Quality Matters: From Clinical Care to Customer Service	available
Practice Management for the Dental Team	Winter 2007

Dental Team, Editor: Mabel Slater

Team Players in Dentistry	Winter 2007

Implantology, Editor: Lloyd J Searson

Implantology in General Dental Practice	available

Quintessence Publishing Co. Ltd., London